HOW TO CHANGE YOUR LIFE WITH RAW & LIVING FOOD

by

Gourmet Raw Food Chef
Sharynne Gambrell-Frazer

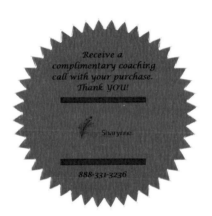

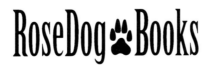

RoseDog❖Books

PITTSBURGH, PENNSYLVANIA 15222

Cover design by
www.alykcreative.com
aly@alykcreative.com
702.862.0238

ISBN: 978-1-4349-9941-2
eISBN: 978-1-4349-5265-3

Printed in the United States of America

First Printing

For more information or to order additional books, please contact:
RoseDog Books
701 Smithfield Street
Pittsburgh, Pennsylvania 15222
U.S.A.
1-800-834-1803
www.rosedogbookstore.com

DEDICATION

This book is dedicated to my beloved mother, Charlice Vincent "Sug" Basey Gambrell, whose compassion for people spearheads this book and is in her memory. She will always be with me.

I love you, Mom!

This book is also dedicated to my dad, George Wellington "Wellie" Gambrell, who has always set such a wonderful example for how to overcome life's challenges. He taught me how to be a pioneer, to live life, and always plan for the future.

I love you and thank you, Daddy-O!

Lastly, I would like to dedicate this book to my very loving, supportive, and always patient husband, Bert. Without you, this book, my dreams, and our goals would not have been possible. You always do whatever is necessary to accomplish my dreams.

I'll love you always, Poppee!

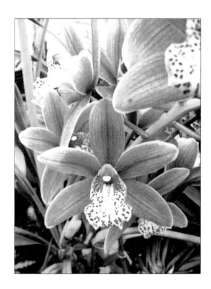

A MESSAGE FROM THE AUTHOR

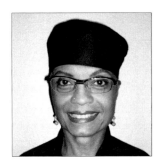 As adults, we know that moment. That 'turning point' in our lives when—sometimes wonderful, sometimes not, but always life-changing—events happen to us. Mine came in July 2005, when my 77-year-old mother was admitted to the hospital. Mom was in her fourth year of dementia, but nothing was wrong, as far as we knew, that threatened her life.

How wrong we were.

More than 40 years of prescription drugs, used to control her high blood pressure, had resulted in polycystic kidney disease, for which there is no cure—the only sign or symptom is sudden death. In fact, within a month, she was dead. Prescription drugs had ravaged her kidneys. Autopsy pictures of them looked like Swiss cheese—the holes allowing toxins to dump directly into her bloodstream, poisoning her.

I was with Mom, Dad and "Binkie", our cat, as I watched, day by day, as she slowly slipped away. One small consolation was that we were able to fulfill a last wish and take her home to be with her family.

Within 36 hours, she was gone.

At some moment during those difficult days and hours—I can't say exactly when—I realized my life was duplicating hers. I, too, had the same medical issues: excess weight, high blood pressure and hand-crippling arthritis. To see myself in her scared me beyond words. But it also marked the 'turning point' I mention above.

Let's skip ahead...

Today my dad is 86 and, except for manageable diabetes, he's in good health. He has a strong fortitude. Since my mother's death, we've added more raw and living food to his diet and have weaned him off sugar. As I'm sure all loving daughters understand, I'm "watching him like a hawk."

For me, the journey into raw food has changed my life, literally. The human body has always been my passion, and with more than 30 years of experience in the medical profession, including the operating room, I know it very well! But since becoming a Gourmet Raw Food Chef and Instructor, I've learned so much more! About:

· Nutrition and how it plays a major role in the quality of our lives.
· Our bodies, and the fact that no matter how badly we abuse them, they have a miraculous ability to heal themselves—sometimes in the form of a repair, sometimes in the form of relief.

I continue to learn, and am now teaching and sharing this passion in my classes.

So, my message to you is this: *If you are currently taking prescription drugs, please read my story carefully, and understand my message...*

There is help for you IF you are willing to take responsibility. There is a whole new world of healthy food and healthy eating waiting for you. And if you choose, it will be a truly wondrous journey of discovery and personal accomplishment!

This is my advice… work with a holistic or naturopath advisor to control your cravings and help you detoxify from refined foods, including meat, dairy and fish. As you detoxify you will notice a dramatic shift in your palate (taste buds). The foods you used to love will not taste as good as before!

For me, the journey into raw food is an evolution that my body has now taken on its own. I have willingly followed, and now experience, health, energy and vibrancy I haven't known since I was in my twenties. Believe it or not, I will be 63 years young on my next birthday!

Listen to your body, it will tell you whether it wants to eat or not. I have learned how to "eat to live," not "live to eat."

With raw food you **DO NOT** starve yourself. Portion control is important, of course, but you will eat delicious and decadent recipes—some so simple they can be prepared in 10 minutes or less.

Decide today to take control of your life, and come join us, please!

Yours in Health!

Chef Sharynne

Contents

FOREWORD

Chef Sharynne Gambrell-Frazer's enthusiasm for her life's work is infectious. As you get to know her, it's easy to believe in and understand her goals for your good health. Her studies are extensive, and she never stops learning and creating.

A woman of the world, Chef Sharynne travels to many areas of our country to spread the word and teach the art of a healthy lifestyle. Enjoy her delicious and healthy recipes in this book. Learn to eat well and live well with *How to Change Your Life with Raw & Living Food.*

I admire Chef Sharynne greatly, as I'm sure you will, too. I'm honored to call her my friend and contemporary.

Karen M. Foster
President/Founder
Las Vegas Now Magazine

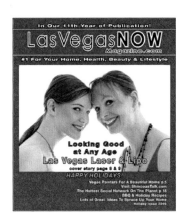

GOURMET RAW FOOD CHEF SHARYNNE GAMBRELL-FRAZER IS A CONTRIBUTING AUTHOR IN THE HIGHLY SUCCESSFUL *WAKE UP...LIVE THE LIFE YOU LOVE*, A BARNES & NOBLE BEST-SELLING BOOK SERIES. THE CHEF SHARES HER PERSONAL STORY OF EMPOWERMENT THAT WAS A RESULT OF A DEVASTATING FAMILY TRAGEDY.

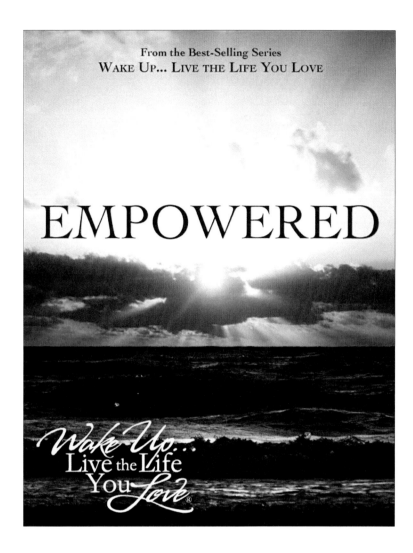

More than fifty writers, mentors, entrepreneurs, and professional leaders have joined Steven E., Dr. Wayne Dyer™, Dr. Michael Beckwith, John Assaraf from *The Secret*, Brian Tracy, Lee Beard, Liz Vassey, Ernie Hudson, and Gregory Scott Reid from the film *Pass it On* to make a difference in your life.

Here are the messages of hope that will encourage you to try again. These stories will light the way to empowerment and a life changed forever. Collectively, they provide the compass that shows the way to permission, authority, and confidence, pointing the way to personal power.

BARNES&NOBLE
BOOKSELLERS

THIS HOUR'S BESTSELLERS

1. Beck, Glenn. *Glenn Beck's Common Sense.*

2. Brown, Dan. *The Lost Symbol.*

3. The Editors, "The Sexy Stars of Twilight," *US Weekly*

4. *E., Steven, et al. *Wake Up...Live the Life You Love: Empowered.*

5. Evanovich, Janet. *Finger Lickin' Fifteen.* Stephanie Plum Series #15.

6. Morris, Dick. *Catastrophe.*

7. Stanton, Doug. *Horse Soldiers.*

8. Meyer, Stephenie. *Twilight Saga Collection.*

9. Gladwell, Malcolm. *Outliers.*

10. Levin, Mark R. *Liberty and Tyranny.*

* *Empowered* hit the BN.com bestseller list in 2009 with the *Wake Up...Live the Life You Love* best-selling series. The book made the number one spot in the Self Improvement category in July and the number four spot in the top 100 list in June.

INTRODUCTION

This book is for very busy people like you.
The majority of the recipes can be prepared in ten minutes or less in real time.
Make quick, easy, and delicious recipes that taste as great as their cooked versions!
Welcome to the world of "Raw and Living Food."
Enjoy!

—Chef Sharynne Gambrell-Frazer

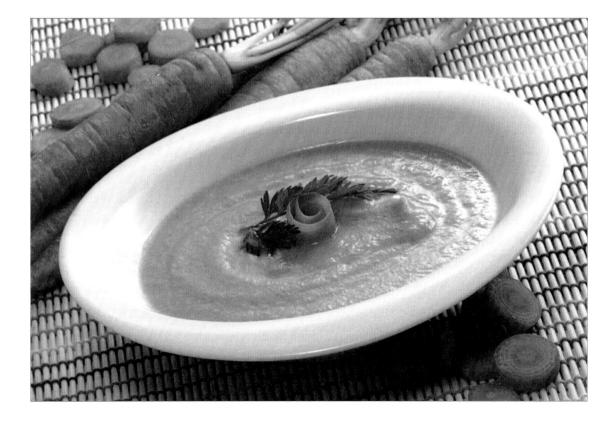

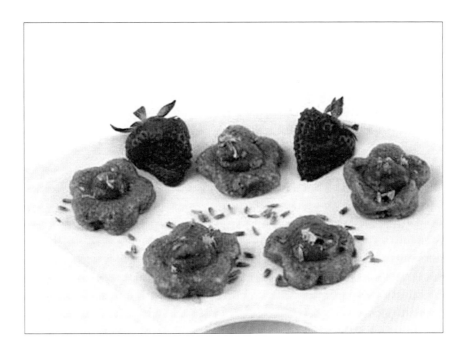

WHAT IS RAW, LIVING, OR WHOLE FOOD?

Raw and living foods are any uncooked fresh fruits, vegetables, nuts, beans, seeds, or sprouted grains. These foods are not heated, cooked, processed, or altered in any way. Raw and living food is nothing more than whole foods in their natural state. The diet of some raw foodists includes raw unpasteurized dairy products such as raw milk, raw meat, raw eggs, and raw honey. Not only can you eat raw fruit, vegetables, nuts, and seeds but you can also sprout grains and beans and eat them, too. This author personally disagrees with any form of animal in your diet. A lifestyle full of animal products will be a life full of disease and illness. There is peer-reviewed science that supports this. (Author T. Colin Campbell, *The China Study*)

WHY IS RAW AND LIVING FOOD HEALTHIER THAN COOKED FOOD?

When food is cooked over 118° Fahrenheit (this temperature can be felt as being warm to the touch), we begin to partially destroy some vital enzymes. This is a problem because we need enzymes for every function of our body. To walk, talk, and move, life itself depends on enzymes. Cooking makes it harder for our bodies to break up and digest the foods we eat. This food then begins to get stored in our bodies as fat (a toxin), which can lead to all kinds of diseases and illnesses, making you more susceptible to **premature death!**

HOW DO I START EATING RAW AND LIVING FOOD?

Just simply start by *eating more fruits and vegetables and reduce the amount of cooked food*. My recommendation is for you to take some classes to educate yourself. Keep an open mind as you experiment and broaden your palate.

Some of my favorite raw and living food recipes are: Pesto-Stuffed Mushrooms, Lasagna, Pizza, Chocolate Macaroon Cookies, Apple Cinnamon Raisin Cookies, and many more. The beauty of the raw-and-living-food lifestyle is that you don't need a lot to get started. We will discuss this later on in the Kitchen Appliances section. You can start by going cold turkey or gradually, whichever you prefer. I highly recommend you see a naturopath or other alternative-healthcare professional before starting, especially if you have medical issues or are taking medications.

WHY WOULD SOMEONE WANT TO EAT RAW AND LIVING FOOD?

The main reason, simply put, is:

Health!

Those who embrace this form of lifestyle invariably experience improvements in their general physical and mental status, including more energy, better health, weight loss, detoxification, and a stronger immune system that resists and recovers from diseases. The list goes on and on.

Many foodists have turned to the raw-and-living-food lifestyle due to medical conditions they faced. They have tried the conventional methods and were getting worse, not better. They asked themselves, What do I have to lose? After all, they could always go back to the prescription drug therapy.

WHERE DO RAW AND LIVING FOODISTS GET THEIR PROTEIN?

The WHO (World Health Organization) says humans need about 5% of their daily calories to come from protein to be healthy. The USDA (United States Department of Agriculture) puts this figure at 6.5%. On average, most fruits have about 5% of their calories from protein.

Vegetables range from 20–25% while sprouted seeds, beans, and grains contain another 10–25%. Therefore, if you are eating a variety of raw and living food, you are getting more than your adequate amount of protein. Numerous scientific studies have shown the daily requirement for protein to be about 25–35 grams a day. Thus, if you eat approximately 2,000 calories a day and ate living foods that averaged about 10% of their calories from protein, you would get 200 calories worth or **50 grams**! This is more than you need on a daily basis.

Other studies have shown that heat-treating a protein (as with cooking) makes about half of it unusable to the human body. There is still this misguided belief that plant protein is not "complete." This is based upon studies done on rats in the 1940s. This conclusion was drawn before we discovered the body's protein-recycling mechanism and its ability to "complete" any amino acid mix from our body's amino acid pool. This false idea is still being perpetuated by the meat and dairy industries in an attempt to influence people to continue consuming their health-destroying products.

IS THIS SOME "NEW FAD DIET" OR SOMETHING?

First of all, this is *no diet*! This is about lifestyle change. Consider this: During the vast majority of our existence on the planet, what choices did we have for food? What *could* we have eaten before we discovered fire, tools, and implements to kill animals? The original diet *must* have consisted primarily of vegetables, fruits, and nuts! What other choices did we have? Clearly, a "raw and living food," plant-based diet is the main food staple throughout the vast majority of the history of mankind! Before we started killing and eating dead animal carcasses, we ate fruits, leaves, nuts, berries, and the like.

"Raw and living food" has gained acceptance in Hollywood with people such as Demi Moore, Cher, Woody Harrelson, Uma Thurman, Susan Sarandon, model Carol Alt, Olympic champion Carl Lewis, recently joining the raw food ranks is John Mackey, CEO of Whole Foods Market, and many more.

IS THIS JUST ANOTHER VEGETARIAN OR VEGAN DIET?

YES and NO. This is the *ultimate* vegetarian/vegan lifestyle. It should be the goal of all vegetarians, vegans, and Standard American Diet eaters to eat raw and living food. Once you embrace this lifestyle change, you will have more energy, better health, improved ability to think more clearly, and become more in tune with your body. This way of eating will last a lifetime and will reward you each and every day of your life.

Is a 100% raw and living food the best?

That depends on the person. I believe life should not be about whether you are eating 100% or 50% raw. It's about your health not an all or none! You can eat "unhealthily," and eat 100% raw and living food and not be eating the correct raw and living food. Start slowly and let your body tell you whether it wants to be 100% raw or not.

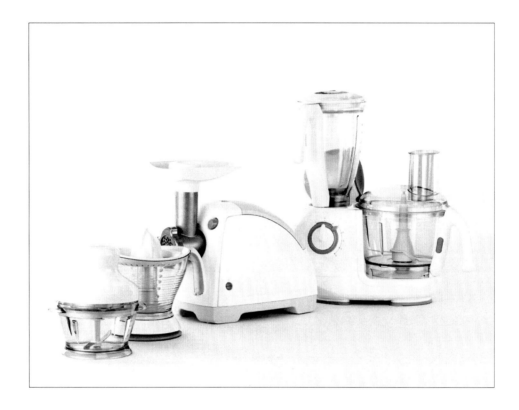

WEEK ONE: KITCHEN AND PANTRY SETUP

Equipment:
- cutting board
- 8-inch chef's knife
- vegetable peeler, spatula, and garlic press
- blender, mandolin, and vegetable spiral slicer
- salad spinner
- Britta water filter (or other water-filter system)

Staples:
- extra-virgin olive oil
- sea salt
- raw almonds, cashews, walnuts
- dates
- dried basil
- dried dill
- onion powder

Add these ingredients to your weekly grocery list:
- fresh fruit
- 3 bananas
- frozen or fresh berries
- 1–2 heads romaine lettuce
- 1–2 heads red leaf lettuce
- 3 avocados
- garlic
- 1 bunch celery
- 2 carrots
- 2 zucchini
- 4 Roma tomatoes
- 1 cucumber

STOCKING YOUR PANTRY (DETAILED)

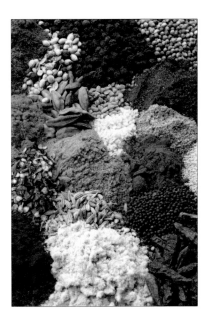

Condiments:
- *ume* vinegar – a pickling by-product from *umbeboshi* plums made with sea salt and *shiso* leaves; ruby red in color, tangy, and very salty.
- sun-dried sea salt
- extra-virgin olive oil – organic, cold-pressed, or, best choice, stone-pressed
- Nama Shoyu – unpasteurized soy sauce (has gluten); San J Organic Tamari - gluten-free
- apple cider vinegar – organic, raw, and unfiltered

Nuts (look for organic, raw, and unsalted):
- macadamia or pine nuts
- cashews or pecans
- almonds, walnuts, and Brazil nuts

Seeds (look for organic, raw, and unsalted):
- sunflower seeds
- sesame seeds (black, beige, and white)
- pumpkin seeds
- hemp seeds
- flax seeds

Nut and Seed Butters (organic, raw, or cold-pressed):
- tahini – smooth butter made from hulled sesame seeds; calcium and protein rich
- coconut butter – a.k.a. "coconut oil"
- cacao butter
- almond, cashew, and macadamia; cashew or peanut *(CAUTION: ALLERGIES)*

Seaweed:
- whole-leaf dulse – whole seed leaf
- *wakame* – tasty, sun-dried seaweed that expands when hydrated
- *nori* – raw is black; toasted is green
- dulse flakes or granules – reddish-purple seaweed rich in alkaline and excellent source of iron, potassium, iodine, and manganese

Spices (look for organic):
- turmeric
- nutmeg
- *garam masala* – Indian word *garam* translates to "warm"; this spice has wide variations of uses in Indian food
- curry powder
- cumin
- coriander
- cinnamon
- chili powder
- cayenne pepper
- black pepper
- apple pie spice

Sweeteners and Dried Fruit (look for organic):
- vanilla bean – use vanilla extract without alcohol; use vanilla bean only when specifically noted as no substitute. Vanilla bean can be costly to your recipe so use sparingly.
- sun-dried tomatoes – source of sulfur dioxide that is generally regarded as safe as per the Consumer Dictionary of Food Additives and the Consumer Dictionary of Cosmetic Ingredients (CDFA), which is a great reference book
- raisins
- mesquite powder – ground ripened mesquite tree seedpods
- lúcuma powder – maple-flavored fruit from Peru; great source of Beta-carotene, Niacin, and Iron
- goji berries – smaller than raisins, contain eighteen amino acids, eight essential amino, and twenty-one trace minerals; it's the richest source of Beta-carotene, 500 times the vitamin C, B_1, B_2, B_6, and E
- dried mango
- dried coconut – unsulphured and unsweetened
- carob powder – look for raw
- agave nectar – light and amber in color; look for raw

Other Foods (look for organic):
- stone-ground mustard
- spirulina – fine powder of blue-green algae with amazing amounts of vitamins, minerals, and phytonutrients, rich in beta-carotene, iron, vitamin B_{12}, and rare, essential fatty acids
- pure water – filtered, distilled, and underwent reverse osmosis, or artesian spring
- maca root powder – root with stamina and libido enhancers, has positive effects on blood pressure (for high or low blood pressure)
- green powder – green food powders, cereal grasses, algae, digestive enzymes from aquatic vegetables, and probiotics (good bacteria)
- Greek olives – look for sun-dried olives cured in sea salt
- cacao nibs or powder

Appliances:
- juicer, preferably Green Star®, Miracle Green Machine®, or Juiceman®
- high-wattage food processor, preferably Cuisinart®, with a three-cup minimum capacity
- economically Hamilton Beach® is the best buy for a food processor in the beginning
- food dehydrator, preferably Excalibur® , 9- or 5-tray
- blender, preferably Vita-mix®, or any high-wattage blender

Nutrition Facts

Serv. Size 1 cup (249g)
Servings About 2
Calories 250
Fat Cal. 110

*Percent Daily Values (DV) are based on a 2,000 calorie diet.

Amount/serving	%DV*	Amount/serving	%DV*
Total Fat 12g	18%	**Sodium** 940mg	39%
Sat. Fat 6g	30%	**Total Carb.** 24g	8%
Polyunsat. Fat 1.5g		Dietary Fiber 1g	4%
Monounsat. Fat 2.5g		Sugars 1g	
Cholest. 60mg	20%	**Protein** 10g	20%

Vitamin A 0% • Vitamin C 0% • Calcium 6% • Iron 8%

INGREDIENTS: WATER, CHICKEN STOCK, ENRICHED PASTA (SEMOLINA WHEAT FLOUR, EGG WHITE SOLIDS, NIACIN, IRON, THIAMINE MONONITRATE [VITAMIN B1], RIBOFLAVIN [VITAMIN B2] AND FOLIC ACID), CREAM (DERIVED FROM MILK), CHICKEN, CONTAINS LESS THAN 2% OF: CHEESES (GRANULAR, PARMESAN AND ROMANO PASTE [PASTEURIZED COW'S MILK, CULTURES, SALT, ENZYMES], WATER, SALT, LACTIC ACID, CITRIC ACID AND DISODIUM PHOSPHATE), BUTTER (PASTEURIZED SWEET CREAM [DERIVED FROM MILK] AND SALT), MODIFIED CORN STARCH, SALT, WHOLE EGG SOLIDS, SUGAR, DATEM, RICE STARCH, GARLIC, SPICE, XANTHAN GUM, CHEESE FLAVOR (PARTIALLY HYDROGENATED SOYBEAN OIL, FLAVORINGS AND SMOKE FLAVORING), MUSTARD FLOUR, ISOLATED SOY PROTEIN AND SODIUM PHOSPHATE.

Baby Food Ingredients?
Learn how to read the labels!

Don't be <u>misled</u>
by product hype and marketing!

How to Read USDA Organic Labels

October 21, 2002, was the first day that organic farmers and processors started to use the U.S. Department of Agriculture (USDA) seal. Use of the seal is strictly voluntary. Very strict and stringent rules and regulations apply in order to qualify for the use of the USDA seal. Farmers will pay approximately $100,000 to $150,000 in fees to the USDA for their use. If farmers gross less than $5,000 from organic products and sell directly to consumers or retailers they are exempted from these requirements. They may call their products "organic," but they can't use the USDA seal.

The USDA has approved four categories of organic labels based upon the percentage of organic content.

1. 100% organic – uses the USDA organic seal

2. Organic – at least 95% of the contents are organic by weight, excluding water and salt (may use the USDA organic seal)

3. Made with organic – at least 70% of the contents are organic; the front product panel may display the phrase "*MADE WITH ORGANIC*" and followed by up to three specific ingredients (may not display the USDA organic seal)

4. Less than 70% of content is organic – may only list those ingredients that are organic on the ingredient panel but may not make any mention of organic on the panel (may not display the USDA organic seal)

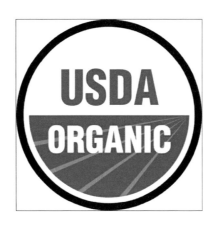

ORGANIC VS. CONVENTIONAL LABELING

Organic food products may optionally display the "USDA Certified Organic" seal. The tiny thumbnail sticker on individual pieces of fresh fruit may have little more than the word "organic" and a product look-up (PLU) code number. The PLU code on organic produce begins with a 9 and is five numbers long (not three or four as with non-organic produce). It's not as good as the USDA Certified Organic certification. However, by checking the PLU code, one is as close as one can come to a double check to see if an item labeled "organic" is actually organic.

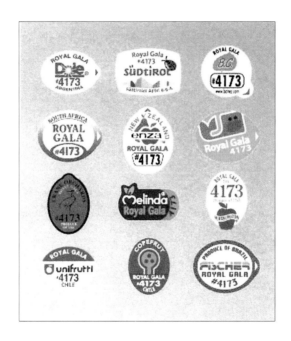

CONVENTIONAL THUMBNAIL STICKERS ON PRODUCE

Have you ever wondered whether the fruit or vegetable you're buying is organic, conventional, or *genetically modified*? Take a look at the PLU that appears on produce stickers.

· Conventionally grown produce stickers are **four digits** long and begin with the numbers **3** or **4**.
· PLU stickers on organically grown produce are **five digits** long and begin with the number **9**.
· PLU codes for genetically modified produce are also **five digits** but begin with the number **8**. You will never see a GMO product label. We will look as this later in "Read the Label" section.

For example, conventional bananas would be code 4011, organic bananas will be 94011, and genetically modified bananas will be 84011.

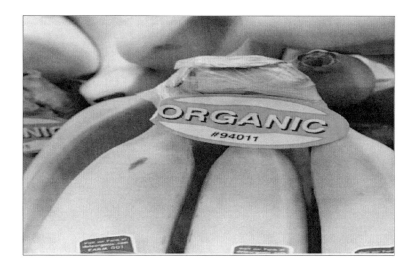

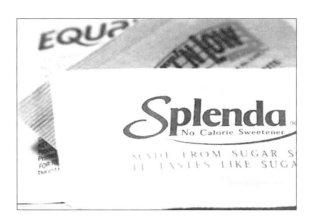

THE FOOD AND DRUG ADMINISTRATION (FDA)
LISTS NINETY-TWO SYMPTOMS FROM NUTRASWEET,
A.K.A. ASPARTAME, INCLUDING DEATH!

Please note: NutraSweet is in Diet Coke, Diet Pepsi, and the majority of sugar-free, low calorie, or no-calorie products.

Article courtesy of: Mark Gold, a researcher for twenty years on such subjects (mgold@tiac.net).
This article originally appeared on www.dorway.com.

Note: This information required a Freedom of Information Act request to pry it from the reluctant hands of the FDA.

NutraSweet (brand name for aspartame) was not approved until 1981, in dry foods. For over eight years, the FDA refused to approve it because of the seizures and brain tumors this drug produced in lab animals. The FDA continued to refuse approval until President Reagan took office (a friend of Donald Rumsfeld, Searle CEO) and fired the FDA commissioner who wouldn't approve it. Dr. Arthur Hull Hayes was appointed new commissioner. Even then, there was so much opposition to approval that a Board of Inquiry was set up. The board said, "Do not approve aspartame," but Dr. Hayes *overruled* his own Board of Inquiry.

Shortly after Commissioner Arthur Hull Hayes, Jr. approved the use of aspartame in carbonated beverages, he left for a position with G.D. Searle's public relations firm.

Long-term Damage. It appears to cause slow, silent damage in those unfortunate enough to not have immediate reactions and a reason to avoid it. It may take one year, five years, ten years, or forty years, but it seems to cause some reversible and some irreversible changes in health over long-term use.

Methanol (a.k.a. wood alcohol/poison composing 10% of aspartame). Methanol/wood alcohol is a deadly poison. People may recall that methanol was the poison that has caused some "skid row" alcoholics to end up blind or dead. Methanol is gradually released in the small intestine when the methyl group of aspartame encounters the enzyme chymotrypsin (a pancreatic enzyme that breaks down protein). The absorption of methanol into the body is sped up considerably when free methanol is ingested. Free methanol is created from aspartame when it is heated to above 86° Fahrenheit (30° centigrade). This would occur when an aspartame-containing product is improperly stored or when it is heated (e.g., as part of a food product such as Jell-O).

Methanol breaks down into formic acid and formaldehyde in the body. Formaldehyde is a deadly neurotoxin. An Environmental Protection Agency (EPA) assessment of methanol states that the substance is "considered a cumulative poison due to the low rate of excretion once it is absorbed." In the body, methanol oxidizes to formaldehyde and formic acid; both of these metabolites are toxic. They recommend a limited consumption of 7.8 milligrams per day. A one-liter (approximately one quart), aspartame-sweetened beverage contains about fifty-six milligrams of methanol. Heavy users of aspartame-containing products consume as much as 250 milligrams of methanol daily, or thirty-two times the EPA limit.

The most well known problems caused by methanol poisoning are vision problems. Formaldehyde is a known carcinogen that causes retinal damage, interferes with DNA replication, and causes birth defects. Due to lack of a couple of key enzymes, humans are many times more sensitive to the toxic effects of methanol than animals. Therefore, tests of aspartame or methanol on animals do not accurately reflect the danger for humans. As pointed out by Dr. Woodrow C. Monte, director of the Food Science and Nutrition Laboratory at Arizona State University, "There are no human or mammalian studies to evaluate the possible mutagenic, teratogenic (the ability to effect the growth and development of an embryo or fetus), [or] carcinogenic effects of chronic administration of methyl alcohol."

It has been pointed out that fruit juices and alcoholic beverages contain small amounts of methanol. It is important to remember that methanol in natural products never appears alone. In every case, ethanol is present, usually in much higher amounts. Ethanol is an antidote for methanol's toxicity to humans. The troops of Desert Storm were treated to large amounts of aspartame-sweetened beverages, which had been heated to over 86° Fahrenheit in the Saudi Arabian sun. Many of them returned home with numerous disorders similar to what has been seen in persons chemically poisoned by formaldehyde. The free methanol in the beverages may have been a contributing factor in these illnesses. Other breakdown products of aspartame, such as dipotassium phosphate (DKP), may also have been a factor.

In a 1993 act that can only be described as *unconscionable*, the FDA approved aspartame as an ingredient in numerous food items that would always be heated to above 86° Fahrenheit (30° centigrade). Much worse, on June 27, 1996, without public notice, the FDA removed all restrictions from aspartame, allowing it to be used in everything, including all heated and baked goods.

The truth about aspartame's toxicity is far different than what the NutraSweet Company would have consumers believe. In February of 1994, the U.S. Department of Health and Human Services released the listing of adverse reactions reported to the FDA (DHHS 1994). Aspartame accounted for more than 75% of all adverse reactions reported to the FDA's Adverse Reaction Monitoring System (ARMS). By the FDA's own admission, fewer than **1%** of those who have problems with something they consumed ever report it to the FDA. This balloons the almost 10,000 complaints they once had to around a million.

The FDA has a history of record-keeping problems. They tend to discourage or even misdirect complaints, at least on the issue of aspartame. The fact remains, though, that *most* victims don't have a clue that aspartame may be the cause of their many problems! Many reactions to aspartame were very serious, including seizures and death.

Those reactions included:

- abdominal pain
- anxiety attacks
- arthritis
- asthma and asthmatic reactions
- bloating or edema (fluid retention)
- blood sugar control problems (hypoglycemia or hyperglycemia)
- brain cancer (pre-approval studies in animals)
- breathing difficulties
- burning eyes or throat
- burning urination
- inability to think straight
- chest pains
- chronic cough
- chronic fatigue
- confusion
- death
- depression
- diarrhea
- dizziness
- excessive thirst or hunger
- fatigue
- feeling unreal
- flushing of face
- hair loss (baldness) or thinning of hair
- headaches/migraines and/or dizziness
- hearing loss
- heart palpitations

- hives (urticaria)
- hypertension (high blood pressure)
- impotency and sexual problems
- inability to concentrate
- infection susceptibility
- insomnia
- irritability
- itching
- joint pains
- laryngitis
- "foggy" thinking
- marked personality changes
- memory loss
- menstrual problems or changes
- muscle spasms
- nausea or vomiting
- numbness or tingling of extremities
- other allergic-like reactions
- panic attacks
- phobias
- poor memory
- rapid heart beat (tachycardia)
- rashes
- seizures and convulsions
- slurring of speech
- swallowing pain
- tremors
- tinnitus
- vertigo
- vision loss
- weight gain

ASPARTAME UPDATE: JANUARY 2010

This article is republished with the express permission of Dr. Mercola in its entirety.

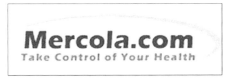

The DVD "Sweet Misery: A Poisoned World" reveals one of the most pervasive, insidious forms of corporate negligence since tobacco. It is an exposé on one of the most deadly chemicals you could find in your food: the artificial sweetener aspartame.

Aspartame products have littered supermarket shelves for almost 30 years, and there are now an estimated 9,000 of them. Aspartame is also a hidden ingredient in many pharmaceutical drugs.

The FDA has received over 10,000 complaints regarding adverse reactions to aspartame. By the FDA's own admission, less than 1 percent of those who experience a reaction to a product ever report it, which translates to roughly a million people who have experienced adverse reactions to aspartame.

A survey conducted by the Calorie Control Council (CCC) reports the following disturbing statistics about current popularity of "low-calorie, sugar-free products" [i]:

- 79 percent of American adults STILL regularly consume low-calorie and sugar-free products, most of which contain artificial sweeteners

- 59 percent of Americans STILL drink diet soft drinks

- 49 percent of Americans STILL use sugar substitutes

If you are one of these statistics, you should watch this film immediately—before you become a FAR GRIMMER STATISTIC. **What you don't know can hurt you.**

THIS FILM CAN LITERALLY SAVE YOUR LIFE

The beautiful aspect of this movie is that, in a short 90 minutes, you will finally understand why aspartame is a toxic poison you need to avoid at all costs.

There are few things you can do in 90 minutes that can make a HUGE impact on your health—but this is one of them.

The toxic long-term effects of aspartame are often dismissed as a "hoax" by the sweetener industry; however this documentary thoroughly unravels truths far more disturbing than any "hoax."

So, grab a tall glass of filtered water and your favorite nutritious snack, plop down in your most comfy chair, and prepare to be blown away.

ONE WOMAN'S NIGHTMARISH ASPARTAME JOURNEY

Part documentary and part detective story, "Sweet Misery" starts with filmmaker and narrator Cori Brackett's poignant story about how she discovered aspartame's ill effects. Brackett had a strange cause-and-effect experience with the diet [colas] she was drinking and quickly found herself disabled and diagnosed with multiple sclerosis.

Her condition quickly progressed to the point that she had double vision, slurred speech, and weak limbs forcing her to use a wheelchair.

When she read an article about aspartame being connected to many health problems, Cori immediately quit using products that contained aspartame—like diet soda.

And magically, many of her symptoms disappeared.

Cori Brackett's journey takes us across the United States to learn more about the devastating effects of aspartame from an impressive list of medical experts—including renowned neurosurgeon Dr. Russell Blaylock, Dr. Betty Martini, two respected physicians and one psychologist.

All experts agreed—aspartame is poison.

STUNNING EVIDENCE OF CORPORATE FRAUD AND MANIPULATION

Aspartame's approval by the FDA may be the most controversial of any food additive in history!

A close examination of the process by which the FDA approved aspartame illustrates how powerful corporations are influencing your once-trusted institutions. In "Sweet Misery" you'll hear this incredible story, featuring:

· Archival footage from G.D. Searle, the producer of aspartame, and federal officials demonstrating the amount of propaganda and "dirty tricks" big business used to push aspartame into the market, including deceptive safety studies.

· Many heart-wrenching testimonials by aspartame victims, including one by a woman serving prison time for murdering her husband, who claims he actually died of aspartame toxicity.

· Key dialogue with Arthur Evangelista, a former Food and Drug Administration investigator, who exposes how far major conglomerates went to legalize the use of aspartame.

· Consumer Attorney Jim Turner's candid report of his exchange with Donald Rumsfeld. Rumsfeld was the CEO of Searle, and at the same time, part of Reagan's transition team when the FDA's board of inquiry was overruled to allow the marketing of aspartame as a food additive. Prior to this time, aspartame was unanimously rejected by the FDA.

A CRASH COURSE IN ASPARTAME TOXICITY

Over the past three decades, aspartame has been associated with multiple neurotoxic, metabolic, allergenic, fetal and carcinogenic effects. Yet it remains a multi-million dollar business today.

Known to erode intelligence and disturb short-term memory, the components of this toxic chemical may lead to a wide variety of ailments.

The following list of health problems are now associated with aspartame consumption:

Brain tumors, including brain cancer. Aspartame can disturb the metabolism of amino acids, protein structure and metabolism, the integrity of nucleic acids, neuronal function and depolarization, and endocrine balance, ultimately leading to tumor growth and cancer. In 1981, an FDA statistician stated the brain tumor data on aspartame was "so worrisome" that he could not recommend approval of aspartame (NutraSweet).

· Leukemia and lymphoma: Two major studies have now confirmed this risk.

· Birth defects: A study funded by Monsanto to look at possible birth defects caused by aspartame was cut off after preliminary data revealed fetal damage.

· A variety of diseases including diabetes, multiple sclerosis, Parkinson's, Alzheimer's, lupus, arthritis, fibromyalgia, and chronic fatigue.

· Emotional disorders like depression[ii], panic attacks, bipolar disorder, and other mental symptoms[iii]. A study from Northeastern Ohio Universities College of Medicine concluded, "[…]individuals with mood disorders are particularly sensitive to this artificial sweetener" and should not use it.

· Epilepsy/seizures: Numerous studies indicate that aspartame makes epilepsy/seizures worse[iv]

· Migraines: 18 million people suffer from migraines, and aspartame may be one of the biggest culprits. Headaches are the most common complaint of aspartame users.

· Numbness

· Hearing loss and tinnitus (ringing in the ears)

· Blindness, blurred vision and other eye problems: More about this in the film "Sweet Misery"—take the time to watch it!

· Stomach disorders

· Heart disease

· Impaired kidney function: A 2009 study found a two-fold increased risk of a decline in kidney function among women who drank two or more artificially sweetened beverages per day.

· Weight gain: Aspartame actually causes you to consume MORE food by tricking your brain into "expecting" some calories, which aren't forthcoming. This results in more cravings and more consumption after you eat or drink aspartame...bad news for your weight loss program!

If you aren't familiar with all the potential health hazards you could be at risk for by consuming this deadly sweetener, "Sweet Misery" will indeed open your eyes to a biomedical genocide that has been covered up for far too long.

If you want more information on aspartame, please check out the collection of articles listed on Dr. Mercola's aspartame page.

Here are some key people, organizations and links mentioned in the film:

· Barbara Martini, Mission Possible World Health International http://www.mpwhi.com/main.htm

· Russell L. Blaylock, M.D. (neurosurgeon) http://www.russellblaylockmd.com/

· Arthur M. Evangelista, PhD. (former FDA Investigator) http://www.wnho.net/articles-aevangelista.htm

· David Oliver Rietz, DORway to Discovery http://www.dorway.com/

· Cori Brackett, blog http://sweetremedyradio.blogspot.com/ and website http://www.sweetremedy.tv/pages/sweetmisery.html

[i] Calorie Control Council http://www.caloriecontrol.org/press-room/trends-and-statistics

[ii] Walton RG, Hudak R, and Green-Waite RJ. "Adverse reactions to aspartame: Double-blind challenge in patients from a vulnerable population" *Biol Psychiatry* 1993 Jul 1-15;34(1-2):13-7 http://www.ncbi.nlm.nih.gov/pubmed/8373935

[iii] Martini B. Letter to the editor of TIME Magazine, http://www.alternativementalhealth.com/articles/aspartame.htm

[iv] "Summary of aspartame-induced seizures issue," Holisticmed.com http://www.holisticmed.com/aspartame/abuse/seizures.html#discussion

ASPARTAME DISEASE MIMICS SYMPTOMS OR WORSENS THE FOLLOWING DISEASES:

· Alzheimer's disease
· arthritis
· birth defects
· chronic fatigue syndrome
· diabetes and its complications
· epilepsy
· fibromyalgia
· lupus
· Lyme disease
· lymphoma
· multiple chemical sensitivities (MCS)
· multiple sclerosis (MS)
· Parkinson's disease

HOW IT HAPPENS

Methanol, from aspartame, is released in the small intestine when the methyl group of aspartame encounters the pancreatic enzyme chymotrypsin. This enzyme is involved in the breakdown of protein (Stegink. 1984, page 143). Free methanol begins to form in liquid aspartame-containing products at temperatures above 86° Fahrenheit, also within the human body.

The methanol is then converted to formaldehyde. The formaldehyde converts to formic acid or ant sting poison. Toxic formic acid is used as an activator to strip epoxy and urethane coatings. Imagine what it does to your tissues!

(*Note from Stephanie Relfe - Kinesiologist*)

(Even the Australian Cancer Council says that there are NO safe levels of formaldehyde).

Phenylalanine and aspartic acid, 90% of aspartame, are amino acids normally used in synthesis of protoplasm when supplied by the foods we eat. But when unaccompanied by other amino acids we use [there are twenty], they are neurotoxic.

That is why a warning for phenylketonurics is found on Equal and other aspartame products. Phenylketonurics are 2% of the population with extreme sensitivity to this chemical unless it's present in food. It gets you by causing brain disorders and birth defects! Finally, the phenylalanine breaks down into DKP (diketopiperazines), **a brain tumor agent!**

In other words, aspartame converts to dangerous by-products that have no natural countermeasures. A dieter's empty stomach accelerates these conversions and amplifies the damage. Components of aspartame go straight to the brain and make damages that cause headaches, mental confusion, seizures, and faulty balance. **Lab rats and other test animals died of brain tumors.**

Despite the claims of Monsanto and bedfellows:

Methanol from alcohol and juices does not get converted to formaldehyde to any significant extent. There is very strong evidence to confirm this fact for alcoholic beverages and fairly strong evidence for juices.

Formaldehyde obtained from methanol is very toxic in *very small* doses, as seen by recent research.

Aspartame causes chronic toxicity reactions/damage due to the methanol to formaldehyde conversion and other broken-down products despite what is claimed otherwise by the very short, industry-funded experiments using a test substance that is chemically different and absorbed differently than what is available to the general public. Strangely enough, almost all independent studies show that aspartame can cause health problems.

A common ploy from Monsanto is to claim that aspartame is "safe," yet a few select people may have "allergic" reactions to it. This is typical Monsanto nonsense, of course. Their own research shows that it does not cause "allergic" reactions. It is their way of trying to minimize and hide the huge numbers of toxicity reactions and damage that people are experiencing from the long-term use of aspartame.

SUMMARY

Given the following points, it is definitely premature for researchers to discount the role of methanol in aspartame side effects:

1. The amount of methanol ingested from aspartame is unprecedented in human history. Methanol from fruit juice ingestion does not even approach the quantity of methanol ingested from aspartame, especially in persons who ingest one to three liters (34-102 ounces or more) of diet beverages every day. Unlike methanol from aspartame, methanol from natural products is probably not absorbed or converted to its toxic metabolites in significant amounts as discussed earlier.

2. Lack of laboratory-detectable changes in plasma formic acid and formaldehyde levels do not preclude damage being caused by these toxic metabolites. Laboratory-detectable changes in formate levels are often not found in short exposures to methanol.

3. Aspartame-containing products often provide little or no nutrients, which may protect against chronic methanol poisoning and are often consumed in-between meals. Persons who ingest aspartame-containing products are often dieting and more likely to have nutritional deficiencies than persons who take the time to make fresh juices are.

4. Persons with certain health conditions or on certain drugs may be much more susceptible to chronic methanol poisoning.

5. Chronic diseases and side effects from slow poisons often build silently over a long period of time. Many chronic diseases that seem to appear suddenly have actually been building in the body over many years.

6. An increasing body of research is showing that many people are highly sensitive to low doses of formaldehyde in the environment. Environmental exposure to formaldehyde and ingestion of methanol (which converts to formaldehyde) from aspartame likely has a cumulative deleterious effect.

7. Formic acid has been shown to slowly accumulate in various parts of the body. Formic acid has been shown to inhibit oxygen metabolism.

8. There are a very large and growing number of persons experiencing chronic health problems similar to the side effects of chronic methanol poisoning when ingesting aspartame-containing products for a significant length of time. This includes many cases of eye damage similar to the type of eye damage seen in methanol poisoning cases.

Note: It often takes at least sixty days without any aspartame NutraSweet to see a significant improvement.
(*Note from Stephanie Relfe: Drink plenty of good water. No tap, distilled, or mineral water*). This author recommends drinking stabilized pH balanced negatively charged alkaline water. (See the chapter on acid/alkaline balance.)
Check all labels very carefully (including vitamins and pharmaceuticals). Look for the word "aspartame" on the label and avoid it. (Also, it is a good idea to avoid "acesulfame-K" or "sunette.") Finally, avoid getting nutrition information from junk food industry PR organizations such as International Food Information Council (IFIC) or organizations that accept large sums of money from the junk and chemical food industry, such as the American Dietetic Association.
If you are a user of any product with aspartame, and you have physical, visual, mental problems, take the sixty-day no aspartame test. If after two months with no aspartame your symptoms are either gone or are much less severe, please become involved to get this neurotoxin off the market. Write a letter to the FDA, with a copy to Betty Martini (for proof of how the FDA doesn't keep proper records). Write your congressmen. Return products containing aspartame to the point of purchase, for a *full* refund. Make a big stink if they *won't* give you a full refund! Tell all your friends and family, and if they stop using aspartame and also "wake up well," get them involved in the same way.
Aspartame is an "approved sweetener" because of a few greedy and dishonest people who place profits above human life and well being. With the FDA and our Congress culpable, only an *informed* and *active* public will affect its reclassification from "food additive" to *toxic drug* and have it removed from the human food chain.

From Stephane Relfe: Note that Michael J. Fox, who was spokesperson for Pepsi, has an old man's disease (Parkinson's disease) at only thirty years old!

Also note: Aspartame has one use that I know of—it makes an *excellent* ant poison. Put a few tablespoons on a nest of fire ants and see how long before they disappear.

FOR MORE INFORMATION:

www.dorway.com
www.aspartamekills.com
www.nexuxmagazine.com/Aspartame.html
http://www.holisticmed.com/aspartame
http://www.trufax.org/menu/chem.html#aspartame

ADDRESSES:

Commissioner
Food and Drug Administration
5600 Fishers Lane
Rockville, Maryland 20857

Mrs. Betty Martini
Mission Possible International
9270 State Bridge Road Suite 215
Duluth, Georgia 30097
E-mail: bettym19@mindspring.com

Now that you are aware of the ninety-two FDA-recognized symptoms (that required a Freedom of Information Act request to pry from their reluctant hands) and *how* aspartame does its dirty work, head to Dorway's Official Dogma page.

www.dorway.com/offasprt.html

On this page, Mark Gold has taken the IFIC "official" aspartame safety myth and shot it full of holes using all of the smoking guns used by the FDA to approve this poison as a food additive, along with information they either ignored or discounted. This excellent debunking of the official FDA/Monsanto/Searle/NutraSweet/NutraSweet Kelco/American Medical Association (AMA)/American Dental Association (ADA)/International Food Information Council (IFIC) chain of lies and half truths, including a long history of this "product's" sordid trail to the marketplace and the sweet tooth.

OTHER GREAT ASPARTAME/PHENYLALANINE LINKS:

www.mercola.com/article/aspartame/phenylalanine.htm
www.heall.com/body/askthedoctor/nutrition/artificialsweeteners.html

EXCITOTOXINS: THE TASTE THAT KILLS
Dr. Russell Blaylock

Excitotoxins are substances added to foods and drinks that literally stimulate nerve cells to death, causing brain damage. They can be found in such ingredients as monosodium glutamate (MSG), aspartame (NutraSweet), and hydrolyzed vegetable protein. The dangers of these substances are so overwhelming that they can no longer be ignored.

Do a search on the web on "aspartame," and you will see that it can cause Parkinson's disease. Why and how did Michael J. Fox, spokesman for Diet Pepsi, get an old man's disease at thirty, multiple sclerosis (MS), and cravings for carbohydrates (thereby causing an *increase* in weight)?

GMOs AND GEs
(Genetically Modified Organisms, Genetically Engineered) Canola, Soybean, Corn, and Cotton . . . Are They?

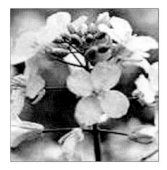 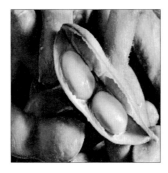 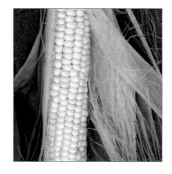 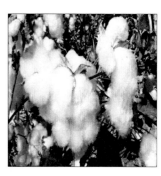

| GM Canola | GM Soybean | GM Corn | GM Cotton |

Consumers have no idea of the number of foods containing GMOs (Genetically Modified Organisms) in their local grocery store. As of today, GMOs don't have to be labeled. In 2006, the *Washington Post* reported that 89% of soybean, 83% of cotton, and 61% of corn are genetically modified in the US. Because of the prevalence of corn and soy in processed foods, *most **Americans have been eating** at **least some GM foods for years, but very few are aware of it.*** In fact, only one quarter of US adults polled believe they have never eaten genetically engineered food.

The body doesn't recognize any modifications made to food due to the manipulation of plant or animal DNA.

Soy: Is It Healthy or Not? What the Experts Say from the WWW.SIXWISE.COM Newsletter

Soy is one of the most widely grown and widely studied legumes in the world (over 5,000 research studies on soy exist). Here in the United States, you are likely familiar with soy in the form of soymilk, soy burgers, soy ice cream, and the myriad of other processed soy products that claim to be ultra healthy.

In truth, studies have shown that certain forms of soy can help to:

· Regulate blood sugar and blood pressure
· Prevent colon, breast, and prostate cancers
· Prevent atherosclerosis (hardening of the arteries)
· Prevent hip fractures in postmenopausal women

Of course, soy wasn't always as popular as it is today. Soy foods have traditionally been considered a "peasant" food, and then a "hippie" food—not something that the average grocery shopper would even consider eating, let alone purposely seek out.

Yet, from 1992 to 2006, soy food sales have increased from $300 million to $3.9 billion according to the Soyfoods Association of North America.

A large part of this increase came when the US Food and Drug Administration (FDA) approved a health claim for soy foods back in 1999 that said:

"Diets low in saturated fat and cholesterol that includes 25 grams of soy protein a day may reduce the risk of heart disease."

Soon after, Americans were clamoring to get their hands on soy in just about every form imaginable. But is it truly healthy?

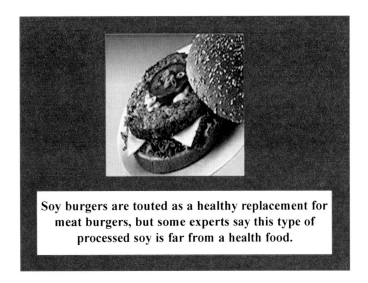

Soy burgers are touted as a healthy replacement for meat burgers, but some experts say this type of processed soy is far from a health food.

Despite findings that soy is good for your heart and your bones and may help to prevent cancer, no public health organization in the United States has recommended a daily intake of soy products, not the National Cancer Institute (NCI), not the American Heart Association (AHA), and not the American Dietetics Association (ADA).

It seems that there is still a lot of conflicting evidence on soy's impact on your body, particularly in the way it is consumed today: processed.

Traditionally, soy in Asian cultures was fermented before eating. This not only makes the beans more digestible, it also increases their nutritive properties while decreasing the presence of phytates, which prevent the absorption of minerals, including calcium, magnesium, iron, and zinc.

Meanwhile, these cultures ate soy in much smaller quantities (about two ounces a day) than Americans now eat soy. If you have a glass of soymilk, you are already drinking more soy than traditional cultures ate in a day. If you add a soy burger and some soy ice cream to that, you are eating an extreme amount of soy, the likes of which has never been consumed in history.

Says Dr. Kaayla Daniel, author of *The Whole Soy Story*:

"Unlike in Asia where people eat small amounts of whole soybean products, western food processors separate the soybean into two golden commodities—protein and oil. There's nothing safe or natural about this.

"Today's high-tech processing methods not only fail to remove the antinutrients and toxins that are naturally present in soybeans but leave toxic and carcinogenic residues created by the high temperatures, high pressure, alkali and acid baths, and petroleum solvents."

In fact, processed soy foods like soymilk, soy meat products, soy ice cream, soy energy bars, etc., have been linked to:

- malnutrition
- digestive problems
- thyroid dysfunction
- cognitive decline
- reproductive disorders
- immune system breakdowns
- heart disease
- cancer

Further, soybeans are one of the most profitable *genetically modified crops* grown in the United States, and they are one of the top eight most allergenic foods.

SOY ISOFLAVONES: A DOUBLE-EDGED SWORD?

Another concern about soy foods has to do with soy isoflavones, which are *phytoestrogens* (estrogens made from plants), a weak form of estrogen that could have a drug-like effect in your body. It is a controversial issue, and some studies suggest that high isoflavone levels might actually increase the risk of cancer, particularly breast cancer.

Daniel Sheehan, Ph.D., director of the Estrogen Knowledge Base Program at the FDA's National Center for Toxicological Research, says isoflavones should be consumed "cautiously."

He says, "While isoflavones may have beneficial effects at some ages or circumstances, this cannot be

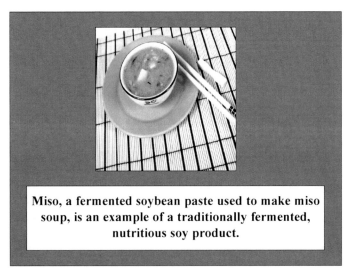

Miso, a fermented soybean paste used to make miso soup, is an example of a traditionally fermented, nutritious soy product.

assumed to be true at all ages. Isoflavones are like other estrogens in that they are two-edged swords, conferring both benefits and risks."

WHICH SOY PRODUCTS *ARE* HEALTHY?

It seems the key to avoiding such health risks when it comes to soy is to stick with only organic unprocessed varieties.

In fact, a study in the June 2004 issue of *Carcinogenesis* found that processed soy products and supplements have a significantly lower ability to prevent cancer and may actually stimulate the growth of preexisting estrogen-dependent breast tumors, compared with whole soy foods.

"These partially purified isoflavone-containing products may not have the same health benefits as whole soy foods," said William G. Helferich, professor of food science and human nutrition at the University of Illinois at Urbana-Champaign and one of the study's lead authors.

Researchers suggested that it may be wise to avoid processed soy products and supplements that contain isoflavones in more purified forms, which is how many Americans consume soy.

Instead, they said to choose minimally-processed whole soy foods.

So, if you're looking for a healthy way to eat and enjoy soy, most experts agree that the following are truly healthy soy options. Always buy organic whenever possible.

- *edamame*
- whole soy flour
- *natto* (fermented soybeans)
- *miso* (fermented soybean paste)
- *tempeh* (fermented soybean cake)
- naturally-fermented soy sauce

Recommended Reading:

"The 6 Healthiest Staple Foods in Japanese Cuisine"
"The Most Dangerous Toxin that Almost No One Knows About"

Sources:

Soyfoods Association of North America
The World's Healthiest Foods

THE TOP 8 FOODS PEOPLE ARE MOST SENSITIVE TO — WITHOUT EVEN KNOWING IT!
Reprinted with permission from the free SixWise.com Security and Wellness e-Newsletter
by Vesanto Melina, MS, RD, and Jo Stepaniak, MS.Ed for SixWise.com

Do you:

- experience occasional or frequent indigestion?
- feel gassy or bloated during meals or shortly after?
- get migraines or other types of headaches?
- frequently have nasal congestion or intermittent joint pain?
- have periodic or seemingly random bouts of anxiety, insomnia, or fatigue?
- **or does your mind sometimes seem foggy?**

Countless people are plagued by these symptoms as well as and an assortment of other ailments that are often misdiagnosed, misunderstood, or brushed off by conventional health care practitioners, leaving us with more questions and confusions than explanations.

Surprisingly, for many individuals, these common complaints may often be linked with a single cause—food sensitivities.

Food sensitivities are broad categories that cover both food allergy and food intolerance.

Food allergy is the reaction of the body's immune system to a food or food ingredient that it recognizes as "foreign."

Food intolerance is an adverse reaction to a food, food ingredient, or additive that does not involve the immune system; it typically involves the digestive system.

Symptoms for both allergies and intolerances can be similar in the skin (e.g. hives or eczema), respiratory system (e.g. asthma), nervous system (e.g. headaches or depression), or digestive tract (e.g. indigestion or bloating).

While almost any food or ingredient might be a trigger for reactions in a few individuals, **the eight culprits responsible for 90% of food reactions are:**

· **milk and milk products**
· **eggs**
· **fish**
· **shellfish**
· **soy**
· **wheat and gluten**
· **peanuts**
· **tree nuts (such as almonds and walnuts)**

Although avoiding a particular food culprit may seem relatively simple, there are many ways we can be exposed to it unknowingly. If we are unusually sensitive, even food particles carried through the air or those that come into contact with our skin may stimulate a reaction. For example (though this situation is rare), peanut aromas have been known to induce a life-threatening response in highly peanut-allergic children.

Cross-contamination, a process whereby particles from a trigger food are introduced to a safe food, is a common occurrence. Cross-contamination can occur during product manufacturing, when several foods are processed on the same factory line, in restaurants when various foods are prepared or served simultaneously, or at home when the same utensil is used to dole out different dishes.

Derivatives from foods we are sensitive to may be "hidden" in prepared products because we may not be familiar with how they are listed on package labels. Or perhaps we just might not be aware of the types of ingredients and food additives that could be causing us difficulty, so we don't know what to be on the lookout for. Sometimes, the solution to a perplexing ailment is as simple as avoiding a single ingredient or adjusting our buying, eating, and kitchen habits to avoid cross-contamination.

If you experience any of these nine health conditions that can be dramatically affected by what you eat, you'll find The Food Allergy Survival Guide to be an indispensable guide!

· arthritis
· asthma
· Attention-Deficit Hyperactivity Disorder (ADHD)
· candida
· dermatitis
· depression
· digestive disorders
· migraines and other headaches

For a complete guide on how to eat if you have food allergies and intolerances, we hope you will consider our new book, *Food Allergy Survival Guide*, which has been highly recommended and is now offered by SixWise.com! You'll learn:

· how to avoid the foods and ingredients that trigger reactions and how to substitute healthful ingredients for those that trigger allergic responses

· how to meet recommended nutrient intakes while avoiding trigger foods such as dairy products, eggs, and gluten-containing grains like wheat or other food culprits

· how food sensitivity may lead to certain ailments such as arthritis, asthma, ADHD (Attention Deficit Hyperactivity Disorder), candida, celiac disease, dermatitis, depression, digestive disorders, fatigue, migraines, and other conditions

· how to determine which food(s) may be triggers for your symptoms

Furthermore, the *Food Allergy Survival Guide* provides 180 pages of delicious recipes that are free of all of the top eight allergens. Read more about the *Food Allergy Survival Guide* now.

Instead of Fritos, Doritos, Cheetos, or Tostitos, Consider *Edamame*
Reprinted with permission from the free SixWise.com Security & Wellness e-Newsletter
by www.SixWise.com

Edamame, the Japanese word for green soybeans, is an integral part of Asian cuisine—one that is becoming increasingly popular with health-conscious Americans. That's because one of the most common ways to enjoy this vegetable is by boiling and salting the pods, then squeezing the beans out for a quick, tasty snack.

While you still won't find *edamame* on the shelves of gas stations like bagged chips, many grocery stores now sell the beans flash-frozen and already salted, so all you need to do is boil them. Or you can grab them completely prepared from a Japanese restaurant if there is one in your area. Point is, when you crave a salty snack, get *edamame*. They're only slightly less convenient than grabbing a bag of chips, but they don't come with the health risks of frying, the negligible nutritional value, or the unsavory additives and preservatives.

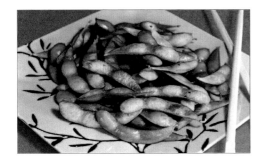

Why *edamame*?

Edamame, which literally means "beans on branches," is quite nutritious. Aside from being high in protein and low in fat, studies have found that isoflavones in soybeans may help:

· reduce the risk of breast cancer in premenopausal women
· decrease the risk of osteoporosis
· promote prostate health
· protect cells with their antioxidant properties

Edamame also qualifies for the FDA-approved health claim for labels of soy foods: *DIETS LOW IN SATURATED FAT AND CHOLESTEROL THAT INCLUDES 25 GRAMS OF SOY PROTEIN A DAY MAY REDUCE THE RISK OF HEART DISEASE* (always look for USDA Certified non-GMO).

Edamame Nutrition Facts

Nutrition	Value	% DV
Serving Size	1/2 cup (75g)	
Amount per Serving	Calories 100	
Amount per Serving	Calories from Fat 25	
Total fat	2.5g	4%
Saturated Fat	0g	0%
Cholesterol	0mg	0%
Sodium	70mg	3%
Total Carbohydrates	0g	0%
Fiber	1g	4%
Sugars	2g	
Protein	10g	

Nutrition	Value	% DV
Vitamin A		10%
Vitamin C		0%
Calcium		8%
Iron		8%

THE HISTORY OF EDAMAME

Edamame may be new in America, but it has been around in China (where it's called *mao dou*) as far back as 200 BC. This is where *edamame* originated, and it was used as a medicinal food. The first recorded use of *edamame* in Japan wasn't until AD 927, when it was described in the *Engishiki*, a guide to agricultural trade. The pods were then used as an offering at Buddhist temples.

DOES SOY PRESENT HEALTH RISKS?

Some believe that soy may not be the health wonder food it's claimed to be. A major aspect of the concern is that soy isoflavones are phytoestrogens, a weak form of estrogen that can have a drug-like effect on the body. It is a controversial issue, and some studies suggest that **high isoflavone levels might actually increase the risk of cancer, particularly breast cancer**.

Daniel Sheehan, Ph.D., director of the Estrogen Knowledge Base Program at the FDA's National Center for Toxicological Research, says isoflavones should be consumed "cautiously." He says, "While isoflavones may have beneficial effects at some ages or circumstances, this cannot be assumed to be true at all ages. Isoflavones are like other estrogens in that they are two-edged swords, conferring both benefits and risks."

It seems the key to avoiding such health risks when it comes to soy is to stick with only unprocessed and non-GMO'd varieties, such as *edamame*, and consume them along with a healthy, varied diet.

In fact, a study in the June 2004 issue of *Carcinogenesis* found that processed soy products and supplements have a significantly lower ability to prevent cancer and may actually stimulate the growth of preexisting estrogen-dependent breast tumors compared with whole soy foods.

"These partially purified isoflavone-containing products may not have the same health benefits as whole soy foods," said William G. Helferich, professor of food science and human nutrition at the University of Illinois at Urbana-Champaign and one of the study's lead authors.

Researchers suggested that it may be wise to avoid processed soy products and supplements that contain isoflavones in more purified forms, which is how many Americans consume soy.

Instead, they said to choose minimally-processed whole soy foods including *edamame*, whole soy flour, tofu, or *tempeh*.

TASTY EDAMAME RECIPES

Edamame can, of course, be eaten plain as a delicious snack, but the beans are so versatile that they can be added to everything, from salads to soups and casseroles. Depending on your nutritional needs, you may want to look for organic or salt-free varieties, all of which can be found in health food stores, Asian markets, and some regular grocery stores.

The University of Kentucky College of Agriculture has put together a free *edamame* cookbook, which has over a dozen unique ways to add *edamame* to your meals at home.

Recommended Reading:

"The Power of the Pomegranate: The 9 Health Benefits of this Wonder Fruit, and How to Eat Them"
"The Healthiest Grasses You Could Possibly Eat (Hint: Not Your Lawn)"

Sources:

FDA: Health Claims for Soy Protein (Internet article)
Kentucky *Edamame* (Internet article)
Edamame: The Vegetable Soybean (Internet article)
The World's Healthiest Foods (book)

This author does not personally support the consumption of *any* form of soybean. This cash cow is another "pulling the wool" over on the public. Soybeans are one of the most profitable seeds in the food chain. Majority of what we eat is genetically modified unless it states non-GMO. The financial potential for corruption is too great.

Food Combining for Health and the Glycemic Index

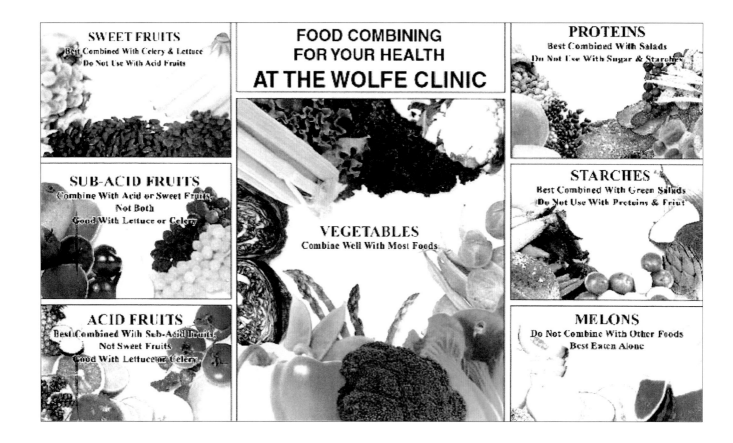

A food-combining diet is based on the principle of separating specific foods and eating them at certain times for good metabolism and proper digestion. This diet has stirred up a lot of disputes among dietitians. Is it really beneficial to health?

Main Principles of Food Combining

Different foods require different digestive conditions. Digestion of food depends on the nutrients in it. Products rich in protein require acidic enzymes for their digestion while those rich in carbohydrates require alkaline enzymes. When acids and alkalis mix in the stomach, they neutralize each other, therefore, worsening and retarding digestion. So, when you eat protein and carbohydrate foods together, some of these nutrients will not be fully assimilated and partly digested food gets into the intestine. As a result, undigested remains deposit as fat and can cause indigestion, bloating, gas, and some diseases. The food-combining diet is pre-ported to resolve the problem.

History

Dr. Herbert M. Shelton is considered to be the founder of the food combining theory. He expounded the key principles of food combining in his works titled *Natural Hygiene or Orthopathy* and *Food Combining Made Easy*. He divided foods into three categories: products rich in protein, products rich in carbohydrates, and the so-called "neutral" products.

Dr. Shelton's basic rules of proper food combining include:

· Eat protein foods and carbohydrate foods at separate meals. They go through different digestive processes.
· Eat acids and starches at separate meals. Acids neutralize the alkaline medium required for digestion of starches.
· Eat fats and proteins at separate meals. Some foods rich in fat (over 50%) require hours for digestion.
· Eat fruits and proteins at separate meals.

Another principle of food combining was suggested by **Dr. Stanley S. Bass** in "Sequential Eating and Food Combining." According to this book, a simple rearrangement of the sequence of foods can improve a person's health. Foods that are digested quickly—for example, fruit—leave the stomach within thirty minutes. If you eat a fruit after a meal, the fruit cannot be digested unless the meal is digested completely. Digesting the meal can take about six or even eight hours. While waiting, the fruit causes the process of fermentation, producing gas and acid. Therefore, Dr. Bass concluded: The most watery food must be eaten first.

FOOD TRANSIT TIMES

water	0–10 minutes	wheatgrass juice	60–90 minutes
juice	15–30 minutes	most vegetables	1–2 hours
rejuvelac	10–15 minutes	grains and beans	1–2 hours
fruit	30–60 minutes	dense vegetable protein	2–3 hours
melons	30–60 minutes	meat and fish	3–4 hours (+)
sprouts	1 hour	shellfish	4–8 hours (+)

IN A NUTSHELL

Dr. Herbert M. Shelton, a prominent American health educator and holistic nutrition advocate, established nine principles for proper food combining. These principles have been reprinted from his book, *Dr. Shelton's Hygienic Review*.

· We should eat acids and starches at separate meals.
· We should eat protein foods and carbohydrate foods at separate meals.
· We should eat but one kind of protein food at a meal.
· We should eat proteins and acid foods at separate meals.
· We should eat fats and proteins at separate meals.
· We should eat sugars (fruits) and proteins at separate meals.
· We should eat sugars (fruits) and starchy foods at separate meals.
· We should eat melons alone. They combine with almost no other food.
· We should desert the desserts. Eaten on top of meals, they lie heavy on the stomach and ferment into alcohols, vinegars, and acetic acids.

CRITICISM

Opponents of the food-combining diet point out that almost all foods are combinations of proteins, carbohydrates, and fats. It is not always easy to classify them strictly into three categories. Besides, the human digestive system is adapted to mixed nutrition and easily copes with different types of food at the same time.

Also, the claim that the food-combining diet helps to lose weight raises a doubt. Opponents believe that those people who prefer this type of diet lose extra pounds because they simply eat fewer calories.

THE BOTTOM LINE

The idea of food combining was discovered at the beginning of the twentieth century and is causing disputes among scientists even in the present time.

On the one hand, the food-combining diet allows eating a variety of foods so you will get the macronutrients (carbohydrates, proteins, and fat), vitamins, and minerals required for good health. It encourages a person to eat more raw fruits and vegetables and less processed foods and added sugars. This principle is also supported by Dietary Guidelines for Americans (DGA), which recommends eating at least five servings of fruits a day.

On the other hand, there is not enough evidence on digestion and weight loss benefits of the diet. In addition, the food-combining diet requires willpower. Following the food-combining diet, you have to eat fish separately from potato or rice. It is not easy to get used to this.

You will usually know if you are a candidate for food combining. Upon eating raw food, you may develop bloating, gas, or a full feeling. Know that the raw food lifestyle should be gradual if you experience any of the above symptoms. Many digestion systems are weak or failing and lack the proper digestive enzymes to break down raw and fibrous foods. This author has no digestive issues and doesn't practice food combining. Yes, you will get the maximum nutrition; however, unless necessary, it can be time consuming.

Take it slowly and gradually introduce more raw food as you develop better enzymes.

References:

Bass, Stanley S., "Sequential Eating and Food Combining."
Bass, Stanley S., "Primitive Man–His Food and His Health."
Shelton, Herbert M. *Orthopathy*.
Shelton, Herbert M. *Food Combining Made Easy*. 1940.
Internet Health Library, "Food Combining"
About.Com, "Food Combining"
United States Department of Health and Human Services. *Dietary Guidelines for Americans, 2005*.

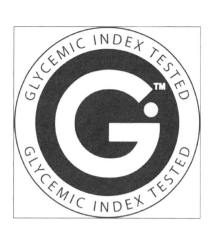

About the Glycemic Index
Article reprinted with permission from the University of Sydney

About Us

Welcome to the "home of the glycemic index," the official website for the glycemic index and international GI database, which is based in the Human Nutrition Unit, School of Molecular and Microbial Biosciences, University of Sydney. The website is updated and maintained by the University's GI Group, which includes research scientists and dietitians working in the area of glycemic index, health, and nutrition, including research into diet and weight loss, diabetes, cardiovascular disease, and PCO (polycystic ovary syndrome), headed by Professor Jennie Brand-Miller. Each month, the Group publishes a free e-newsletter, *GI News*, to bring consumers and health professionals up to date with the latest GI research from around the world.

The GI (glycemic index) is a ranking of carbohydrates on a scale from 0 to 100 according to the extent to which they raise blood sugar levels after eating. Foods with a high GI are those which are rapidly digested and absorbed and result in marked fluctuations in blood sugar levels. Low-GI foods, by virtue of their slow digestion and absorption, produce gradual rises in blood sugar and insulin levels and have proven benefits for health. Low GI diets have been shown to improve both glucose and lipid levels in people with diabetes (type 1 and type 2). They have benefits for weight control because they help control appetite and delay hunger. Low GI diets also reduce insulin levels and insulin resistance. This index is the basis of Nutrisystems® weight loss programs.

Recent studies from Harvard School of Public Health indicate that the risks of diseases such as type 2 diabetes and coronary heart disease are strongly related to the GI of the overall diet. In 1999, the WHO (World Health Organization) and FAO (Food and Agriculture Organization) recommended that people in industrialized countries base their diets on low-GI foods in order to prevent the most common diseases of affluence, such as coronary heart disease, diabetes, and obesity.

Measuring the GI

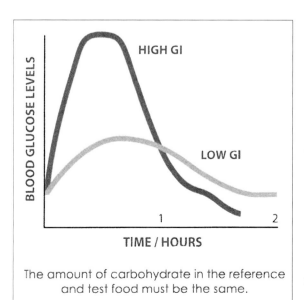

The amount of carbohydrate in the reference and test food must be the same.

To determine a food's GI rating, measured portions of food containing 10–50 grams of carbohydrate are fed to ten healthy people after an overnight fast. Finger-pricked blood samples are taken at fifteen- to thirty-minute intervals over the next two hours. These blood samples are used to construct a blood sugar response curve for the two-hour period. The AUC (area under the curve) is calculated to reflect the total rise in blood glucose levels after eating the test food. The GI rating (%) is calculated by dividing the AUC for the test food by the AUC for the reference food (same amount of glucose) and multiplying by 100 (see Figure 1). The use of a standard food is essential for reducing the confounding influence of differences in the physical characteristics of the subjects. The average of the GI ratings from all ten subjects is published as the GI of that food.

The GI of foods has important implications for the food industry. Some foods on the Australian market already show their GI rating on the nutrition information panel. Terms such as complex carbohydrates and sugars, which commonly appear on food labels, are now recognized as having little nutritional or physiological significance. The WHO/FAO recommends that these terms be removed and replaced with the total carbohydrate content of the food and its GI value. However, the GI rating of a food must be tested physiologically, and only a few centers around the world currently provide legitimate testing service.

The Human Nutrition Unit at the University of Sydney has been at the forefront of glycemic index research for over two decades and has tested hundreds of foods as an integral part of its program. Jennie Brand-Miller is the senior author of "International Tables of Glycemic Index" published by the American Journal of Clinical Nutrition in 1995 and 2002.

Glycemic Index Symbol Program

The GI Symbol Program was launched in Australia in 2002 to help consumers identify the GI of foods. Foods that carry the symbol are guaranteed to have been properly tested by an accredited laboratory.

In the near future, many more foods are likely to carry the GI on their nutrition panel.

The services of a professional GI testing service such as SUGiRS will therefore allow food companies to take advantage of GI marketing opportunities.

GLYCEMIC INDEX FOOD CHART

LOW GI (LESS THAN 55)—GREEN
INTERMEDIATE GI (BETWEEN 55 AND 70)—BLUE
HIGH GI (MORE THAN 70)—RED

FOOD LIST	RATING	FOOD GLYCEMIC INDEX
Bakery Products		
*Pound cake	Low	54
Danish pastry	Medium	59
Muffin (unsweetened)	Medium	62
Cake, tart	Medium	65
Cake, angel	Medium	67
Croissant	Medium	67
Waffles	High	76
Doughnut	High	76
Beverages		
Soya milk	Low	30
Apple juice	Low	41
Carrot juice	Low	45
Pineapple juice	Low	46
Grapefruit juice	Low	48
Orange juice	Low	52
Biscuits		
Digestives	Medium	58
Shortbread	Medium	64
Water biscuits	Medium	65
Ryvita	Medium	67
Wafer biscuits	High	77
**Rice cakes	High	77
Breads		
Multi grain bread	Low	48
Whole grain	Low	50
Pita bread, white	Medium	57
Pizza, cheese	Medium	60

FOOD LIST	RATING	FOOD GLYCEMIC INDEX
Hamburger bun	Medium	61
Rye-flour bread	Medium	64
Whole meal bread	Medium	69
White bread	High	71
White rolls	High	73
Baguette	High	95

Breakfast Cereals

All-Bran	Low	42
Porridge, non instant	Low	49
Oat bran	Medium	55
Muesli	Medium	56
Mini Wheats (wholemeal)	Medium	57
Shredded Wheat	Medium	69
Golden Grahams	High	71
Puffed wheat	High	74
Weetabix	High	77
Rice Krispies	High	82
Cornflakes	High	83

Cereal Grains

Pearl barley	Low	25
Rye	Low	34
Wheat kernels	Low	41
Rice, instant	Low	46
Rice, parboiled	Low	48
Barley, cracked	Low	50
Rice, brown	Medium	55
Rice, wild	Medium	57
Rice, white	Medium	58
Barley, flakes	Medium	66
Taco Shell	Medium	68
Millet	High	71

Dairy Foods

Yogurt low-fat (sweetened)	Low	14
Milk, chocolate	Low	24
Milk, whole	Low	27
Milk, Fat-free	Low	32
Milk, skimmed	Low	32
Milk, semi-skimmed	Low	34
*Ice-cream (low-fat)	Low	50
*Ice-cream	Medium	61

Fruits

Cherries	Low	22
Grapefruit	Low	25
Apricots (dried)	Low	31
Apples	Low	38
Pears	Low	38
Plums	Low	39
Peaches	Low	42
Oranges	Low	44
Grapes	Low	46
Kiwi fruit	Low	53

FOOD LIST	RATING	FOOD GLYCEMIC INDEX
Bananas	Low	54
Fruit cocktail	Medium	55
Mangoes	Medium	56
Apricots	Medium	57
Apricots (tinned in syrup)	Medium	64
Raisins	Medium	64
Pineapple	Medium	66
**Watermelon	High	72

Pasta
Spaghetti, protein enriched	Low	27
Fettuccine	Low	32
Vermicelli	Low	35
Spaghetti, whole wheat	Low	37
Ravioli, meat filled	Low	39
Spaghetti, white	Low	41
Macaroni	Low	45
Spaghetti, durum wheat	Medium	55
Macaroni cheese	Medium	64
Rice pasta, brown	High	92

Root Crop
Carrots, cooked	Low	39
Yam	Low	51
Sweet potato	Low	54
Potato, boiled	Medium	56
Potato, new	Medium	57
Potato, tinned	Medium	61
Beetroot	Medium	64
Potato, steamed	Medium	65
Potato, mashed	Medium	70
Chips	High	75
Potato, microwaved	High	82
Potato, instant	High	83
**Potato, baked	High	85
Parsnips	High	97

Snack Food and Sweets
Peanuts	Low	15
*M&Ms (peanut)	Low	32
*Snickers bar	Low	40
*Chocolate bar; 30g	Low	49
Jams and marmalades	Low	49
Crisps	Low	54
Popcorn	Medium	55
Mars bar	Medium	64
*Table sugar (sucrose)	Medium	65
Corn chips	High	74
Jelly beans	High	80
Pretzels	High	81
Dates	High	103

Soups
Tomato soup, tinned	Low	38
Lentil soup, tinned	Low	44

Food List	Rating	Food Glycemic Index
Black bean soup, tinned	Medium	64
Green pea soup, tinned	Medium	66
Vegetables and Beans		
Artichoke	Low	15
Asparagus	Low	15
Broccoli	Low	15
Cauliflower	Low	15
Celery	Low	15
Cucumber	Low	15
Eggplant	Low	15
Green beans	Low	15
Lettuce, all varieties	Low	15
Low-fat yogurt, artificially sweetened	Low	15
Peppers, all varieties	Low	15
Snow peas	Low	15
Spinach	Low	15
Young summer squash	Low	15
Tomatoes	Low	15
Zucchini	Low	15
Soya beans, boiled	Low	16
Peas, dried	Low	22
Kidney beans, boiled	Low	29
Lentils green, boiled	Low	29
Chickpeas	Low	33
Haricot beans, boiled	Low	38
Black-eyed beans	Low	41
Chickpeas, tinned	Low	42
Baked beans, tinned	Low	48
Kidney beans, tinned	Low	52
Lentils green, tinned	Low	52
Broad beans	High	79

Notes:

*high in empty calories
**low-calorie and nutritious foods

COSMETICS

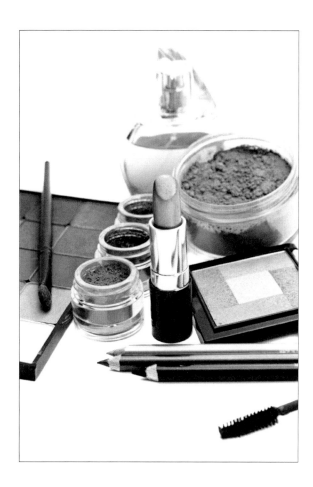

LAW AND REGULATIONS

Major loopholes in U.S. federal law allow the $50 billion cosmetics industry to put unlimited amounts of chemicals into personal care products with no required testing and no monitoring of health effects and inadequate labeling requirements. In fact, cosmetics are among the least-regulated products on the market.

This section explores what's being done to change the broken U.S. system, and how other countries are leading the way to smarter laws that protect their citizens.

The Food and Drug Administration (FDA) does not review, nor does it have the authority to regulate, what goes into cosmetics before they are marketed to salons and consumers.

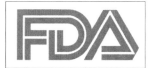

FDA REGULATIONS

The agency charged with oversight of cosmetics, the U.S. FDA has no authority to require pre-market safety assessment as it does with drugs, so cosmetics are among the least-regulated products on the market. The FDA does not review, nor does it have the authority to regulate, what goes into cosmetics before they are marketed for salon use and consumer use. In fact, 89% of all ingredients in cosmetics have not been evaluated for safety by any publicly accountable institution.

Ironically, most American consumers believe the U.S. government regulates the cosmetics industry the same way it regulates food and drugs sold in this country to make sure they're safe. The truth is, no one's minding the store when it comes to shampoo, skin moisturizers, baby products, lipsticks, or any other personal care product.

The FDA's own web site explains its limitations:

> "FDA's legal authority over cosmetics is different from other products regulated by the agency. Cosmetic products and ingredients are not subject to FDA premarket approval authority, with the exception of color additives."

The emerging evidence on the body burdens of chemicals in the American people, as well as the new science on how small exposures to these chemicals can add up to harm, suggests that there is no health-based rationale for the difference in regulatory powers among the different FDA divisions.

According to the FDA, "[a] change in FDA's statutory authority over cosmetics would require Congress to change the law." To discourage congressional legislation, the cosmetics industry trade group (then the Cosmetic, Toiletry, and Fragrance Association and now the Personal Care Products Council) created a system of voluntary self-regulation in 1976 through the Cosmetic Ingredient Review panel.

THE FOX GUARDING THE HEN HOUSE

The Cosmetics Ingredients Review (CIR), the industry's self-policing safety panel, falls far short of compensating for the lack of FDA oversight. According to its web site, the CIR "thoroughly reviews and assesses the safety of ingredients used in cosmetics in an open, unbiased, and expert manner, and publishes the results in the peer-reviewed scientific literature."

Yet, in its more than thirty-year history, the CIR has reviewed the safety of only 11% of the ingredients used to formulate personal care products, and through June of 2008 has found only nine ingredients to be unsafe for use in cosmetics.

This panel operates in a vacuum of guidance from FDA when it comes to the safety of personal care products. Words on labels like "natural," "safe," and "pure" have no definition in law and no relationship to the hazard inside the packaging. Acceptable levels of risk are entirely at this panel's discretion.

To the detriment of public health, the CIR doesn't look at the effects of exposures to multiple chemicals linked to negative health impacts, the cumulative effect of exposures over a lifetime, and the timing of exposure, which can magnify the harm for the very young and other populations or worker exposures in both beauty salons and manufacturing plants.

Voluntary self-regulation of the cosmetics industry in the United States is not working. Consumers deserve a government that protects them from unsafe chemical exposures in the cosmetics they use every day.

In order to achieve real oversight on cosmetics by the FDA, Congress must change existing federal law.

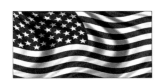

FEDERAL LEGISLATION

The U.S. Federal Food, Drug, and Cosmetic Act (FDCA) is a set of laws passed by Congress in 1938, giving authority to the FDA to oversee the safety of those products. Chapter VI of the FDCA governs the way the massive cosmetic industry is regulated in the United States—and it's all only about two pages long.

Over its seventy-year history, there have been only two attempts to strengthen the federal oversight and regulation of the cosmetics industry: first in 1973, by Missouri Senator Thomas Eagleton, and then in 1988, by Oregon Representative Ron Wyden. Both attempts were unsuccessful because of strong industry lobbying against the measures. It's no wonder the industry is opposed to change in Congress. According to the FDA, "[a] change in FDA's statutory authority over cosmetics would require Congress to change the law."

The Campaign for Safe Cosmetics supports efforts to change federal law and mandate the FDA to exert real authority over the safety of personal care products. While some companies are working toward safer products today, and we applaud those efforts, it shouldn't be up to individual consumers to figure out what's safe and what's not.

In the absence of federal oversight, states have taken steps to ensure that consumers have access to safer cosmetics and more information about the products they buy.

STATE LEGISLATION

Numerous states have introduced safe cosmetics legislation over the last four years. Two notable successes are:

· Washington State adopted legislation in 2008 that bans phthalates from personal care products marketed to or used by kids, part of the broader Children's Safe Products Act.

· In 2005, California became the first state in the nation to pass state legislation governing the safety and reporting of cosmetic ingredients. The California Safe Cosmetics Act requires manufacturers to disclose to the state any product ingredient that is on state or federal lists of chemicals that cause cancer or birth defects.

STATUS UPDATE

California is in the process of collecting ingredient information from cosmetics manufacturers now, pursuant to the 2005 law. We expect the data to be published in early 2009 on a publicly accessible database.

WHAT YOU CAN DO...

If you're interested in passing safe cosmetics laws in your state, contact mia@safecosmetics.org for resources and information.

EUROPEAN LAW

The European Union has more stringent and protective laws for cosmetics than the United States. Now twenty-five countries strong, the EU has tougher and more protective laws for cosmetics than the United States. The hazard-based, precautionary approach of the EU acknowledges that chemicals linked to cancer and birth defects simply don't belong in cosmetics—regardless of the concentration of the chemical being used.

The United States has much to learn from the EU's example. The EU Cosmetics Directive (76/768/EEC) was revised in January 2003 to ban 1,100 chemicals from cosmetics; the U.S. FDA has banned or restricted only eleven.

That means that companies are no longer allowed to sell personal care products in the European Union that are made with chemicals that are known or suspected to cause cancer, genetic mutation, reproductive harm, or birth defects. The Compact for Safe Cosmetics expands on the EU laws and asks companies to commit to removing the EU-banned chemicals from products sold in the United States and elsewhere around the world.

The European Union is also proposing to change the way it regulates all chemicals in order to better protect human health. The EU wants to require chemical companies to test chemicals for health effects before they are put on the market, but the Bush Administration worked to stop Europe from passing these protective laws. See this report by Rep. Henry Waxman for more information on U.S. interference with the EU plan to change the way chemicals are regulated:

http://www.safecosmetics.org/downloads/Waxman-report_2004.pdf

American consumers deserve the same protection as our neighbors in Europe. However, without the force of law, nothing is stopping U.S. cosmetic companies from producing a safer product for distribution in the EU and a toxic product to sell back home. The United States needs to ramp up its protection of consumers and adopt stronger federal oversight and regulation of chemicals linked to adverse health effects in cosmetics and personal care products sold in the U.S. and globally.

More Information:
European Commission: Cosmetics Directive (consolidated; multiple languages):
http://ec.europa.eu/enterprise/sectors/cosmetics/files/doc/cons_simpl/effci_en.pdf

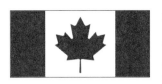

CANADIAN LAWS

The Canadian government recently created a Cosmetic Ingredient Hotlist that includes hundreds of prohibited and restricted chemicals and contaminants. Canadian cosmetics regulations, like European Union Regulations, are stricter than those in the United States. The Canadian government recently created a Cosmetic Ingredient Hotlist that includes hundreds of prohibited and restricted chemicals and contaminants such as formaldehyde, triclosan, selenium, nitrosamines and 1,4-dioxane—all of which are allowed in U.S. products.

In addition, cosmetic manufacturers are required to register their products and disclose a list of ingredients and the concentration of each ingredient used. Labeling requirements that went into effect in November 2006 in Canada require ingredient lists to appear on all cosmetic product labels. Increased disclosure is making choosing safe products easier for Canadian consumers.

According to the Health Canada Web site, "only ingredients that do not pose an unreasonable health and safety risk to the Canadian public, when used according to directions, are allowed in cosmetic products."

More Information
Health Canada: Cosmetic Ingredient "Hotlist":
http://www.hc-sc.gc.ca/cps-spc/person/cosmet/info-ind-prof/_hot-list-critique/hotlist-liste_1-eng.php

THE FDA AND LEAD IN LIPSTICK

More than a year after promising to conduct an analysis of lead in lipstick, the FDA has released no information to the public. After the Campaign for Safe Cosmetics released the 2007 report, "A Poison Kiss: The Problem of Lead in Lipstick," which found lead in popular lipstick brands, the FDA promised to conduct its own analysis of lead in lipsticks, but it took two years for the FDA to release its information to the public despite pressure from U.S. senators and repeated calls from health groups, including letters from the Campaign for Safe Cosmetics.

The FDA published its long-awaited study on lead in lipstick in the July/August 2009 issue of the Journal of Cosmetic Science. The article is available only through the Journal's web site for a cost of $35 and does not name the brands or shades it tested. The FDA study did, however, find lead in all lipsticks it tested, and at higher levels than we found in 2007.

Why the holdup? The FDA said it was waiting for a peer-reviewed journal to publish its study of lead in lipstick. This delay tactic kept a taxpayer-funded study from the public for nearly two years.

In fact, the FDA used similar delaying tactics to bury information about phthalates in personal care products. In July 2002, an independent analysis by members of the Campaign for Safe Cosmetics found that 72% of personal care products tested contained phthalates, a set of industrial chemicals linked to reproductive harm. FDA conducted its own study of phthalates in personal care products in 2003 but did not release the data to the public despite an Freedom of Information Act (FOIA) request submitted by Campaign for Safe Cosmetics partner, Friends of the Earth.

The FDA study was finally published three years later in a scientific journal not available for free to the public.

About the Campaign for Safe Cosmetics

The Campaign for Safe Cosmetics is a coalition of women's, public health, labor, environmental health, and consumer rights groups. Our goal is to protect the health of consumers and workers by requiring the health and beauty industry to phase out the use of chemicals linked to cancer, birth defects, and other health problems. We are asking the industry to replace them with safer alternatives.

Personal care products like shampoo, conditioner, aftershave, lotion, and makeup are not regulated by the FDA or any other government agency. It is perfectly legal and very common for companies to use ingredients that are known or suspected to be carcinogens, mutagens, or reproductive toxins in the their products. Consumers buy these products at drug stores, grocery stores, online, or in salons, usually without questioning the product's safety.

We are asking cosmetics and personal care products companies to sign the Compact for Safe Cosmetics (also known as the Compact for the Global Production of Safer Health and Beauty Products), a pledge to remove toxic chemicals and replace them with safer alternatives in every market they serve. As of August 2007, 600 companies have signed the Compact—and that number increases every day!

The Campaign works with endorsing organizations and individuals so that, together, we can ramp up the pressure on companies that have not signed the Compact and continue to sell us toxic products, including Estee Lauder, L'Oreal, Avon, and many others.

Our founding organizations also work closely with other allies to reform the chemical policies that allow toxic ingredients in consumer products in the first place.

HISTORY OF THE CAMPAIGN

The Safe Cosmetics Campaign began in 2002 with the release of a report, "Not Too Pretty: Phthalates, Beauty Products, and the FDA." For the report, environmental and public health groups contracted with a laboratory to test seventy-two brand name, off-the-shelf beauty products for the presence of phthalates, a family of industrial chemicals linked to permanent birth defects in the male reproductive system.

The lab found phthalates in nearly three-quarters of the products tested, though the chemicals were not listed on any of the labels. A second report, "Pretty Nasty," documented similar product test results in Europe.

In February 2003, the European Union passed a new amendment to their Cosmetics Directive that prohibits the use of known or suspected CMRs (carcinogens, mutagens, and reproductive toxins) from cosmetics. This amendment went into force in September 2004.

FOUNDING GROUPS OF THE CAMPAIGN FOR SAFE COSMETICS INCLUDE:

Alliance for a Healthy Tomorrow, Breast Cancer Fund, Clean Water Fund, Commonweal, Environmental Working Group, Friends of the Earth, Massachusetts Breast Cancer Coalition, National Black Environmental Justice Network, National Environmental Trust, and Women's Voices for the Earth.

In spring 2004, these groups and more than fifty other organizations signed a letter asking cosmetics companies to take their pledge, the Compact for Safe Cosmetics. Today, 600 companies have signed the Compact.

Together, we are working for safer products and smarter laws that will protect our health and our families from toxic chemicals.

If your nonprofit organization would like to support our efforts, please email us for our newsletter: info@safecosmetics.org.

What is the Acid/Alkaline Balance?

The pH Scale Is from 0–14

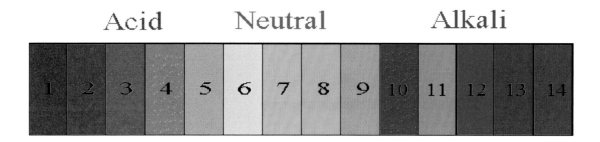

Human blood pH should be slightly alkaline (7.325–7.425). Below or above this range means symptoms and disease. A pH of 7.0 is neutral. A pH below 7.0 is acidic. A pH above 7.0 is alkaline. An acidic pH can occur from acid-forming diet, emotional stress, toxic overload, and/or immune reactions or any process that deprives the cells of oxygen and other nutrients. The body will try to compensate for acidic pH by using alkaline minerals. If the diet does not contain enough minerals to compensate, a build up of acids in the cells will occur.

An acidic balance will decrease the body's ability to absorb minerals and other nutrients, decrease the energy production in the cells, decrease the body's ability to repair damaged cells, decrease the body's ability to detoxify heavy metals, make tumor cells thrive, and make the body more susceptible to fatigue and illness. A blood pH of 6.9, which is only slightly acidic, can induce coma and death.

The reason acidosis is more common in our society is mostly due to the typical American diet, which is far too high in acid-producing animal products like meat, eggs, and dairy and far too low in alkaline-producing foods like fresh vegetables. Additionally, we eat acid-producing processed foods like white flour and sugar, and we drink acid-producing beverages like coffee and soft drinks. We use too many drugs, which are acid forming, and we use artificial chemical sweeteners like NutraSweet®, Spoonful®, Sweet 'N Low®, Equal®, or aspartame, which are poisons and extremely acid forming.

One of the best things we can do to correct an overly acidic body is to clean up our diet and lifestyle.

To maintain health, diet should consist of 60% alkaline-forming foods and 40% acid-forming foods. To restore health, diet should consist of 80% alkaline-forming foods and 20% acid-forming foods.

Generally, alkaline-forming foods include most fruits, green vegetables, peas, beans, lentils, spices, herbs and seasonings, and seeds and nuts.

Generally, acid-forming foods include meat, fish, poultry, eggs, grains, and legumes.

WATER FACTS

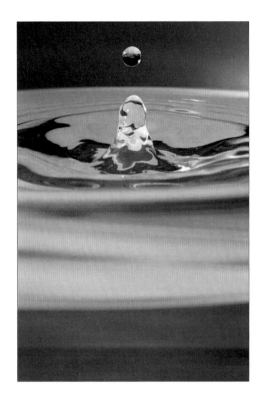

ABOUT pH AND ORP

Ionized alkaline drinking water is saturated with negatively charged ions. These negatively charged ions attract the positively charged ions of harmful acids and neutralize them. Scientists have devised ways to measure and assign values to the electron activity. The measurement is known as ORP or oxidative reduction potential.

ACIDITY IN THE BODY

The human body creates acid all day, each and every day, as a by-product of metabolism. In addition, acid is introduced into the system through eating and digestion. Many secreted and digested acids are swept away by the blood stream, filtered out by the kidneys, and released from the body in the urine. Other acids leave the body through perspiration. Your body can only process a certain amount of acids, however, so it is possible to overload the system and for the body to become acidity.

ALKALINE WATER BENEFITS

The ionization process breaks down water molecules into micro-clusters, allowing rapid delivery to cell walls for a superior hydrating effect at a cellular level. Micro-clustered water delivers nutrients to the cells more efficiently. Among several other benefits, including proper hydration, detoxification, and balance in your body's pH levels, drinking alkaline water can ultimately contribute to weight loss and anti-aging.

HYDRATION

Hydrated cells are healthy cells. A well-hydrated cell absorbs oxygen and nutrients and disposes toxins and wastes efficiently. Dehydrated cells are inefficient cells. Unfortunately, thirst is not an accurate guide to the body's hydration levels. By the time you feel thirsty, you already are dehydrated.

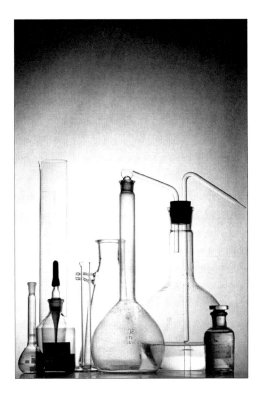

WHAT IS ACIDIC WATER?

Acidic water (often referred to as electrolyzed water) is water with a potential hydrogen (pH) of less than 7. The pH level refers to the amount of hydrogen mixed in with the water. The pH level is measured on a scale of 0 to 14; 7 represents "neutral," where the water is neither alkaline nor acidic; 0 through 7 indicates acidity, and 7 through 14 indicates alkalinity.

Signs of acidic water:

- blue stains on copper fixtures or pipes
- blue or green stains in tubs or basins
- pH test showing less than 7 is considered acidic
- a sharp or chlorine smell at the tap

Home water sources have been known to have a pH level of less than 5.5, which many water treatment solutions will not guarantee service for or offer systems to deal with.

Like the Richter scale for measuring earthquake intensity, the pH scale is logarithmic. A solution with a pH of 8.0 is ten times more alkaline than a solution with a pH of 7.0. A solution with a pH of 9.0 is 100 times more alkaline than a solution with a pH of 7.0.

The intake of **acidic water**, along with the acidic foods in the modern diet, causes the body to work overtime to maintain the blood pH within the health range. To do so, the body will take alkaline substances from body parts such as bones. By drinking alkaline water, a person is able to reduce the intake of acids and increase the availability of alkaline minerals, helping the body regulate its pH in a healthier way.

Recent studies of **acidic water** uses have discovered many home uses. For example, a recent patent in Europe has been filed after a study showing **acidic water** obtained by electrolysis is a highly effective treatment of dermatosis in domestic animals when applied or sprayed several times at the initial stages of the dermatosis.

Medical and dental offices often use acidic water to destroy microorganisms as well as a sterilizing hand wash.

ALKALINE WATER BENEFITS

Restores the pH balance in the body (The body's pH is alkaline in nature ranging from 7.325-7.425.):

- Alkaline water can neutralize the acidity of the body caused by stress, modern diet, air pollution, and many bottled waters.

- A higher pH in the body reduces the need for fat and cholesterol to protect the body from damaging acids.

- Alkaline water is negatively charged and an antioxidant. Antioxidants reduce cellular and DNA damage caused by free radicals.

- Negatively charged alkaline water creates energy by giving up ions to positive ions.

- Alkaline water tastes lighter, with a pleasantly sweet flavor.

- Using water with a higher pH level improves the taste of beverages and food.

· Cooking with alkaline water improves the taste and quality of foods, and using acidic water when boiling eggs improves their quality.

Provides superior hydration and nutrition at the cellular level:

· Ionization breaks clusters of water molecules into smaller microclusters, reducing the size of the clusters from the eleven to sixteen molecules in standard water to just five to six molecules in ionized water. Smaller clusters pass through cell walls (referred to as semi-permeable membrane) more easily and hydrate the cells more quickly.

· Faster hydration allows the body to regulate its temperature more efficiently.

· Microclusters of mineral-bearing ionized water also deliver nutrients more efficiently to the cells.

Detoxifies cells more efficiently than standard drinking water:

Due to their smaller size, microclusters of ionized water molecules are expelled from the cells more efficiently, carrying damaging toxins out of the cells and flushing them out of the system. The negative charge of ionized alkaline water will attract the positive ions of acids and neutralize them within the body.

There are several versions of the Acidic and Alkaline Food chart to be found in different books and on the Internet. The following foods are sometimes attributed to the acidic side of the chart but sometimes to the alkaline side. Remember, you don't need to adhere strictly to the alkaline side of the chart; just make sure a good percentage of the foods you eat come from that side.

Brazil nuts	maple syrup
Brussels sprouts	milk
buckwheat	nuts
cashews	organic milk (unpasteurized)
chicken	potatoes, white
corn	pumpkin seeds
cottage cheese	quinoa
eggs	sauerkraut
flaxseeds	soy products
green tea	sprouted seeds
herbal tea	squashes
honey	sunflower seeds
kombucha	tomatoes
lima beans	yogurt

Chef Sharynne is an authorized Life Ionizer Dealer: www.lifeionizer.com/chefsharynne

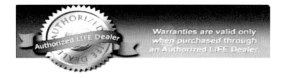

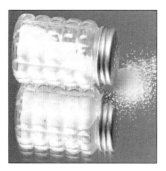
Table Salt

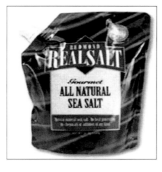
All Natural Sea Salt

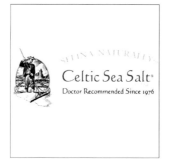
Celtic Sea Salt ® Brand

Coarse Himalayan Salt

Regular table salt starts out as a saline solution. After processing and kiln drying at high temperatures in excess of 400° F all the trace minerals are destroyed. Chemicals like Silica aluminate, Potassium iodide, Tri-Calcium Phosphate, Magnesium Carbonate, Sodium Bicarbonate, and yellow prussiate of soda are added to bleach out the salt and prevent caking, thus allowing free flowing even on rainy days. Back in the day your mother may have added dry rice or popcorn kernels to the salt shaker before there were chemicals!

Perchlorate, a component of rocket fuel, has leaked out of military sites and contaminated the drinking water in many states. It has been found in foods, and cow's milk. According to the Centers for Disease Control (CDC) Perchlorate has been found in 1 out of 3,000 people tested. One third of women tested with lower Iodine levels when exposed to Perchlorate. It's been found in food and the environment. This is very troublesome for women of childbearing age because of the developing fetus that is vulnerable to decreases in the maternal thyroid hormone.

Himalayan Salt is composed of natural elements such as Nitrogen, Beryllium, Boron, Magnesium, Silver, Palladium, Iodine, Rubidium and Nickel—all the elements our bodies need to function properly. Salt is one of the essential elements for electrical impulses and general conductivity within the body.

Salt has long been used in homeopathic medicine and has been used for centuries to combat symptoms and illnesses. Himalayan Salt has been used as part of dental hygiene to prevent bleeding gums and bad breath, as an ear infection remedy, to lessen acne, combat foot fungus, alleviate psoriasis, soothe sore throats, lessen headaches and neck pain and balance the body's natural pH. Natural crystal salt can now be found in many lotions, bath salts and skin care products.

CAUTION: Himalayan salt may contain high levels of Fluoride. Check with your healthcare practitioner before using.

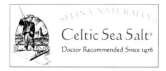
WHY CELTIC SEA SALT® BRAND?
(Printed with full permission of Celtic Sea Salt® Brand)

<u>Because it's "Dr Recommended"...</u>

Celtic Sea Salt® Brand Sea Salts contain a higher percentage of mineral-dense natural brine (sea water). This bio-available high moisture content naturally lowers the amount of Sodium Chloride found in our salts. Hand-harvested, unrefined Celtic Sea Salt® Brand Sea Salts are recommended by Doctors and Natural Health Practitioners around the world. Our "Sea the Difference" chart below demonstrates the natural trace mineral and moisture content found in several sea salts available at local supermarkets.

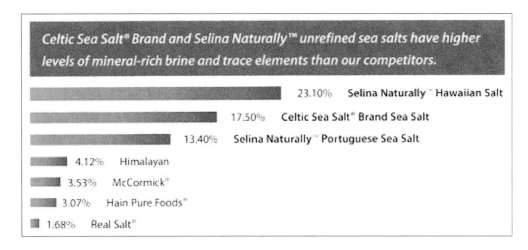

Celtic Sea Salt® Brand and Selina Naturally™ unrefined sea salts have higher levels of mineral-rich brine and trace elements than our competitors.

23.10%	Selina Naturally™ Hawaiian Salt
17.50%	Celtic Sea Salt® Brand Sea Salt
13.40%	Selina Naturally™ Portuguese Sea Salt
4.12%	Himalayan
3.53%	McCormick®
3.07%	Hain Pure Foods®
1.68%	Real Salt®

Sea water contains natural trace minerals such as ionized Sodium, Magnesium, Calcium, Potassium, and Selenium, plus trace elements such as Copper, Iron, Zinc, Manganese, and Chromium. The human body uses these minerals and trace elements to create electrolytes, and maintain bodily fluids. This "internal ocean" is vital to the proper functioning of every system within our body.

The distinctive moisture of Celtic Sea Salt® Brand Sea Salt is mineral-rich brine, or "Mother Liquor," that has been traditionally used for centuries as a health elixir. Naturally formed sea salt crystals are saturated in this life giving "Mother Liquor." Celtic Sea Salt® Brand Sea Salt is hand-harvested and carefully packaged to preserve the integrity of this phenomenal union.

With hundreds of Doctors and Natural Health Practitioners recommending Celtic Sea Salt® Brand Sea Salt worldwide, it is no wonder that our product continues to receive industry and consumer praise alike. Health Professionals recommend Celtic Sea Salt® Brand Sea Salt as a natural alternative to refined salt that may help balance blood pressure while enhancing the flavor and quality of foods.

The Original Brand™ is the most trusted brand. Celtic Sea Salt® Brand is referenced in more culinary and nutritional books and journals than any other salt in the world.

· known to help balance blood pressure
· great for hypertension
· better for diabetics
· contains no added chemicals/anti-caking agents
· contains all of the minerals of the ocean, not just NaCl
· Doctor recommended

Celtic Sea Salt® Brand salt is authentic, unprocessed whole salt from one of the most pristine coastal regions of France. Since 1976, Celtic Sea Salt® Brand salt has been harvested by the paludiers (salt farmers) of Brittany using a farming method that preserves the purity and balance of ocean minerals. Our Celtic Sea Salt® is certified organic by Nature and Progres, the highest level of certification allowed in France.

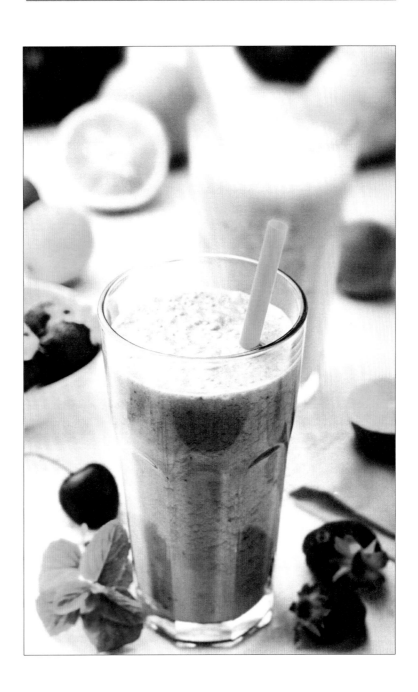

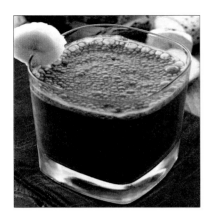

GREAT FOR THE BONES SMOOTHIE
Serves 1–2

2 bananas
1 c soaked and sprouted brown sesame seeds
2 c nut milk
2 tbs cacao powder
a drop of vanilla (alcohol free)

Blend until smooth.

CHEF SHARYNNE'S OREO SMOOTHIE
Serves 1–2

juice of 1 coconut (or container of coconut water)
2 tbs soaked almonds
1 tbs raw cacao nibs or powder
organic sweetener to taste (optional)
1/2 soft vanilla bean snipped into small pieces with scissors

Blend until smooth.

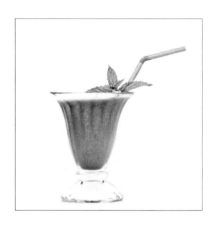

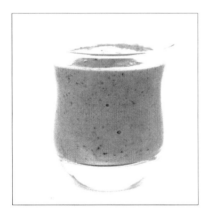

CHERRY BABY CASHEW SMOOTHIE
Serves 1–2

1 1/2 c cashew milk (2 parts water to 1 part nuts if you want to make your own)
1 1/2 c frozen cherries
1 c frozen sliced banana
1 tbs vanilla
organic sweetener (optional)
a pinch of sea salt
variation: add 1/2 tsp ground cinnamon

Blend until smooth.

CHEF SHARYNNE'S HOLIDAY SMOOTHIE
Serves 1–2

4 c almond or oat milk
2/3 c raw macadamia nuts
8 soft-pitted dates or raisins
2 bananas, peeled and frozen
2 tsp vanilla
2 tsp nutmeg

Blend all, except banana, in blender till smooth. Add bananas and blend. Sprinkle with nutmeg and serve.

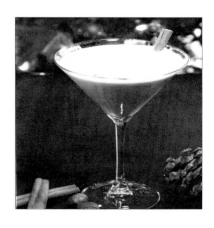

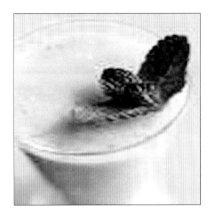

Oh, Oh, Orange Cream Smoothie
Serves 1–2

1 c almond or cashew milk (2 parts water to 1 part nuts)
1 orange, peeled, seeded (not juiced, just the whole orange)
1 frozen banana, cut up
optional: 2 dates or raisins
several ice cubes

Blend until smooth.

Popsicle Smoothie
Serves 3–5

2 c crushed ice
2 c pineapple, fresh or frozen
3 c freshly-squeezed orange juice
2 c strawberries, fresh or frozen
1 large banana
1 mango

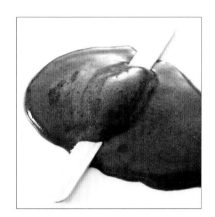

Chill a large glass in the freezer while you are preparing the smoothie. Process all ingredients in a blender until smooth. <u>Add the crushed ice after</u> all the fruits have been blended. Remove your glass from the freezer. They should be frosty in appearance by then. Pour your smoothie into your glass.

<u>Note</u>: If you want a thicker smoothie, then cut back on the orange juice to 2 c. If you want it thinner, then just add more orange juice. Seasonal fruits make an excellent choice for this smoothie. They can all be easily substituted. Omit using the crushed ice during the summer; just pour them into Popsicle molds and freeze. This is a real kid favorite!

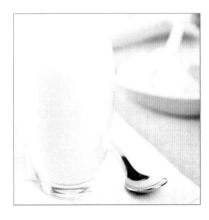

Pineapple Princess
Serves 1–2

1 handful of kale or Swiss chard
1 c fresh pineapple
2 bananas
1 c orange juice
1–2 c nut milk, apple juice, water or ice

Blend until smooth.

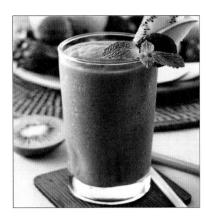

MANGO MADNESS
Serves 1–2

1 small handful of parsley
1–2 mangoes
1 c orange juice
1–2 c nut milk, apple juice, water or ice

Blend until smooth.

Old Blue Eyes
Serves 1–2

1 large peach or 2–3 small peaches
1 c frozen blueberries
1/2 cucumber
lots of spinach

Blend until smooth.

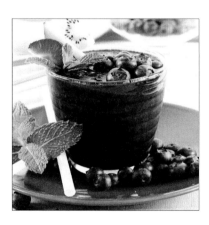

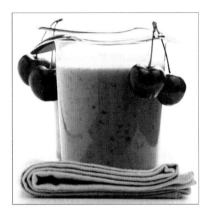

Cherry Baby
Serves 1–2

2 c nut milk, apple juice, water or ice
1/2 avocado (ripe)
2 bananas
1/2 bag of spinach
1 bag of frozen cherries
organic sweetener (optional)

Blend until smooth.

This smoothie is great for controlling cravings!

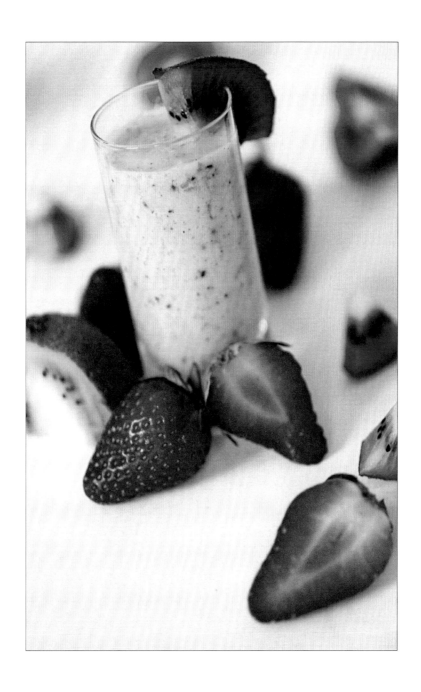

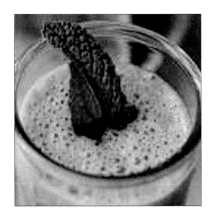

POPPEE THE SAILOR MAN
Serves 1–2

1/2 apple
1 orange
1 c packed spinach
1 tbs cacao beans
1/4 c frozen blueberries
1 tbs flaxseed
organic sweetener (optional)
garnish: kiwifruit and strawberry (optional)

Blend until smooth.

LETTUCE ENTERTAIN YOU!
Serves 1–2

6–7 bananas
4 peaches
romaine lettuce
1/4 c nut milk, apple juice, water or ice

Blend until smooth.

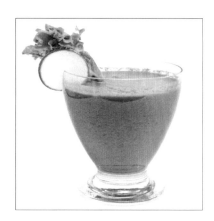

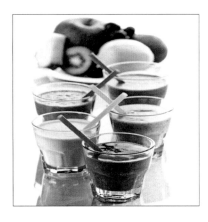

MOCHA PASSION
Serves 1–2

1/2 apple
1 orange
1 c packed spinach
1 tbs cacao beans
1/4 c frozen blueberries
1 tbs ground flaxseed
organic sweetener to taste (optional)

Blend until smooth.

KBOP (KALE, BANANA, ORANGE, AND PINEAPPLE)
Serves 2–3

1 handful of kale or Swiss chard
1 c fresh or frozen pineapple
2 bananas
1 c orange juice
1–2 c nut milk, apple juice, water or ice
organic sweetener to taste (optional)

Blend until smooth.

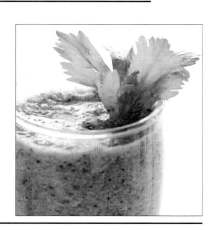

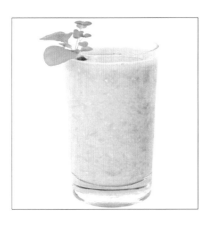

PARMANGO
Serves 2–3

1 small handful parsley
1–2 mangoes
1 c orange juice
1–2 c nut milk, apple juice, water or ice
organic sweetener to taste (optional)

Blend until smooth.

STRAWBERRY GREENS FOREVER
Serves 2–3

1 handful of greens (any kind)
2 c strawberries
2 bananas
1–2 c ice or water
organic sweetener to taste (optional)

Blend until smooth.

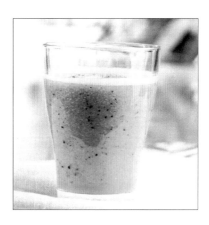

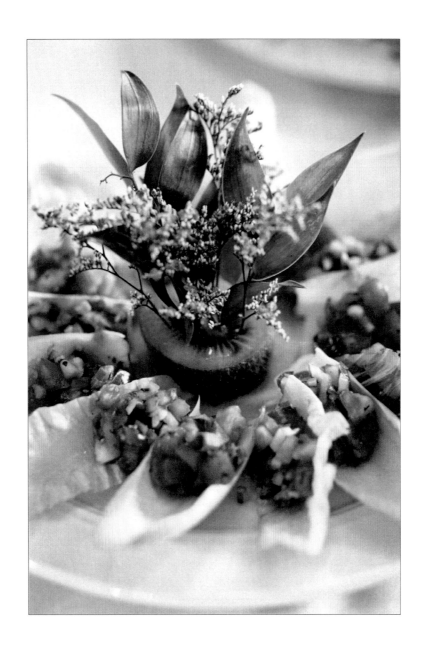

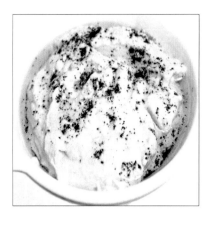

HUMMUS – HOLD THE BEANS
Serves 1-2
A delicious, thick, beanless hummus.

2 ea zucchini, peeled and chopped
3/4 c raw tahini
1/2 c fresh lemon juice
1/4 c extra-virgin olive oil
4 ea cloves garlic, peeled
2 1/2 tsp sea salt
1/2 tbs ground cumin

In a high-speed blender or food processor, combine all ingredients and blend until smooth and thick. Yummy!

Serving suggestions: Serve this with cayenne pepper, sesame seeds, and paprika. You can substitute lime juice for lemon. Instead of zucchini, you can substitute with cucumber slices or red or yellow bell pepper.

SUMMER CORN OFF THE COB SALAD
Serves 4–6
Organic sweet corn off the cob, diced celery, and scallions are lightly tossed and drizzled in a creamy sauce.

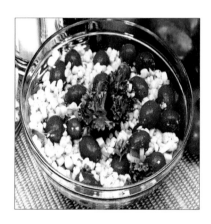

The Salad
3 c fresh corn kernels (approximately 4 ears of corn)
1 c coarsely-chopped celery
1 c chopped scallions (green onions)
1 bunch fresh parsley, stems removed; cilantro, destemmed; or dill
1 ea tomato, red and yellow peppers, and carrots (*optional*)

The Dressing
1/2 c nut milk, purified water, or coconut water
1/4 c fresh lemon juice
organic sweetener to taste
2 tbs extra-virgin olive oil
1 1/2 tsp sea salt
3/4 tsp curry powder, or to taste
1/4 c raw pine nuts
1/2 avocado (optional, if you want the dressing to be creamy)

In a large mixing bowl, combine all salad ingredients and toss, mixing it thoroughly. In a high-speed blender or food processor, combine all of the dressing ingredients and blend until smooth. Pour over the salad and toss well to mix the dressing with the corn, and serve.

Additional options: radishes, red onion, mango, lime juice, cayenne, or chipotle

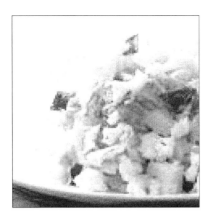

CAULIFLOWER: IS IT A FLOWER SALAD?
Serves 4–6

2 c diced cauliflower
1 c corn
1/2 c sliced radishes
1/2 c diced red, yellow, and green peppers
1/2 c diced celery
2 unpeeled red apples, diced
1/4 c parsley
3 sliced scallions (green onions)

The Dressing
2 tbs pine nuts
1/4 c coconut water, coconut milk, or nut milk
1 tbs lemon juice
1/8 tsp hot sauce (optional)

Prepare vegetables as directed and toss together with dressing; serves 4–6. Additional options: zucchini, purple onion, orange bell peppers, raisins, cranberries, pistachios, carrots, and cherry tomatoes for garnish.

CUCUMBER AND ONION SALAD
Serves 1–2

1 cucumber, sliced
1 small to medium onion (I prefer red), sliced
3/4 c red wine vinegar
1/2 c water
organic sweetener to taste
1/4 tsp mustard seed
1/8–1/4 tsp each of sea salt and coarse ground pepper

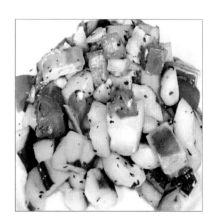

In a medium bowl, separate onions into rings and add to cucumber slices. Add agave nectar to wine vinegar, mustard seed, sea salt, and pepper. Pour over cucumbers and onions and toss. Add diced tomatoes (optional). Allow to marinate for at least an hour before serving.

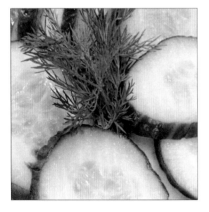

CUCUMBER-DILL SALAD
Serves 2–3

5 cucumbers, peeled and sliced thinly (coring cucumber extends refrigeration)
1 small- to medium-sized onion (I prefer red), sliced
2 bunches fresh dill, chopped and stems removed

The Dressing
1/2 c raw apple cider vinegar
1/2 c extra-virgin olive oil
1/4 c orange juice
1/4 c lemon juice
1–1 1/2 tbs organic sweetener
3/4 tsp sea salt

In a large bowl, combine all salad ingredients. Toss to mix thoroughly. In a food processor, combine dressing ingredients and blend until smooth. Pour over the salad, mix well, and serve.

DESSERTS

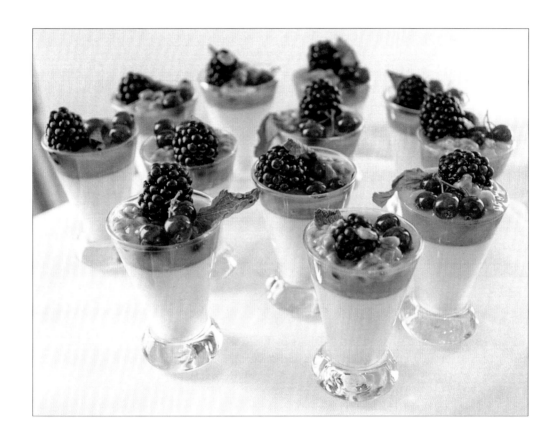

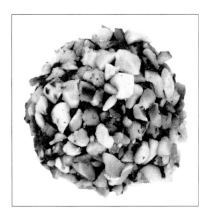

CHEF SHARYNNE'S ALMOND DELIGHT
Makes 12–24 balls
I whipped this up one night by mistake! How sweet it is.

2 c almonds
1 c raisins
1 tsp vanilla
1–3 tsp organic sweetener to taste
shredded unsweetened coconut (optional)
lemon or orange zest (optional)

Add all ingredients in a food processor. Mix well and form into balls. We like them refrigerated and cold; otherwise, it's up to you! If you like a lot of crunch, then pulse-chop this mixture to desired chunky texture. You can roll in shredded coconut, unsulfured and unsweetened (optional), carob, or chopped nuts.

"L" IS FOR LEMON COCONUT BARS
Makes 12 bars

1 c chopped almonds
1 1/2 c soaked and pitted dates (Medjool)
1 tbs vanilla extract
1/2 tbs sea salt
zest of 1 lemon (For a lighter lemon flavor, use Meyer lemons.)
juice of 1 lemon (approximately 2 tbs)
1 c shredded coconut, unsulfured and unsweetened (optional)

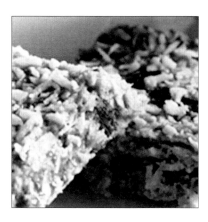

In a food processor, chop almonds into small pieces. In a mixing bowl, add remaining ingredients, including the remaining chopped almonds. Press into a baking pan.
Chill for a couple of hours until firm, then cut into squares. These will last for six days in a refrigerator. You can also roll them into coconut balls for a higher recipe yield.

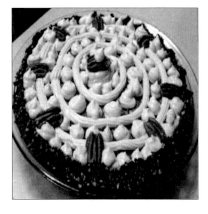

ADAM'S APPLE PIE WITH WALNUT AND CASHEW CREAM TOPPING
Serves 6–8
This is a raw, fresh apple pie made with any combination of Granny Smith, Fuji, and Delicious apples or a single type of apple.

Crust:
2 c almonds
2 tbs organic sweetener
1 c raisins
1/2 tsp sea salt

Process the almonds and the sea salt together until you get a dry almond meal (do not overprocess). Add the agave and raisins, pulse-chop just enough to incorporate them until it is well mixed. It will look like coarse wet sand.

Press mixture into a pie dish. Press firmly into the bottom and sides, smoothing it out. Chill in the fridge to set while you make the filling.

Filling:
4–5 large apples
1 tbs lemon juice
1 tsp ground cinnamon

Cashew Cream Topping:
Makes about 2 1/4 c thick or 3 1/2 c regular cream

2 c whole raw cashews (Do not use pieces, which are often dry), rinse **well under cold water**
1-2 tsp alcohol-free vanilla
1 tsp fresh squeezed lemon juice
organic sweetener to taste (optional)
1/4 tsp freshly-grated nutmeg

Pulse-chop the apples in a food processor. In a large mixing bowl, toss apples with the cinnamon and nutmeg. Spoon the apple mixture into chilled pie crust. Smooth out and garnish with chopped walnuts.

BLUEBERRY HILL CHEESECAKE
Serves 4–6
A very, very sweet and blueberry-flavored cheesecake—with no guilt! You can substitute any of the listed fruits such as kiwifruit, strawberries, mangoes, peaches, blackberries, or mixed berries, and top it with raw whipped cream.

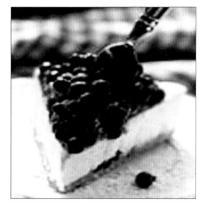

Crust:	Filling:
2 c almonds	4 c cashews
1 c raisins	1 large lemon, juiced
	8–10 tbs organic sweetener
	2 1/2 tsp vanilla
	2 c blueberries or substituted fruit (may be frozen)

For Crust:

Place the almonds in a food processor and blend until fine. Add raisins and blend until well blended. Pat crust down into a glass pie plate. If sticky, moisten fingers with water or fruit juice. Make crust as firm and compacted as possible. This will help to hold form when cutting slices. A good crust will also aid in removing slices from plate. Chill in the refrigerator while making the filling.

For Filling:

Place the cashews, agave, vanilla, lemon, and blueberries in a food processor or blender and process until smooth and creamy. Remove this mixture from the food processor or blender. Pour filling into crusted plate. Chill or freeze for approximately thirty to forty-five minutes for faster set up.

Note: The filling can be made in the food processor but will be creamier if you use a Vita-Mix or a strong blender. Soaking the cashews for a few hours or up to thirty-six hours will help to make this creamier if you're using a food processor.

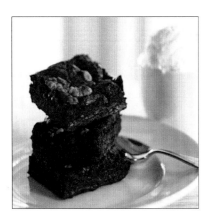

WALNUT FUDGE
Makes 12–24
Mmmmmm, Mmmmmm, Mmmmmm, Mmmmmm, Mmmmmm!

2 c walnuts
1/4 c dates, soaked and pitted
2 tbs organic sweetener
1 tsp cinnamon

Grind walnuts in food processor until fine. Add remaining ingredients and blend until creamy. Fold in additional chunks of walnuts (optional). Form into balls or a large block and keep in refrigerator.

BREAKFAST

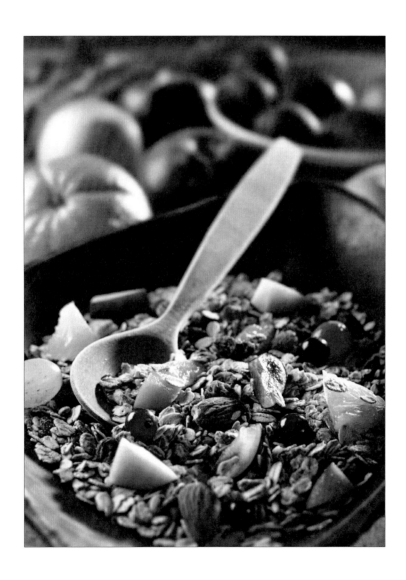

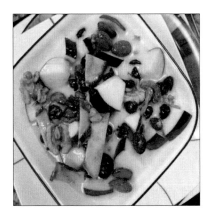

BREAKFAST MUESLI GOOD MORNING
Serves 1–2
A real quick, delicious, and easy breakfast or snack muesli.

2 apples or peaches (fresh or dried)
1/2 c dried organic cranberries
1/4 c flaxseeds, brown or golden
1/4 c organic raisins
1/3 c raw cashews, almonds, and walnuts
2 rehydrated or fresh pears (preferably Asian)
organic sweetener (optional)

Place all the above ingredients in a bowl. Add almonds, oat, and rice milk and enjoy. (You can make your own rice milk or purchase.) Add organic sweetener to taste.

Note: Strawberries, blackberries, or any fruit may be substituted. For additional flavor, presoak the nuts in cooled chai tea. Let nuts air dry or dry in dehydrator. Nuts may be stored in a glass jar in the refrigerator 3-5 days.

COCONUT CHAI BREAKFAST CAKE
Serves 1–2
A lightly-spiced cake with chai flavor, lightly sweet, and very dense, it's perfect for breakfast and great for a snack!

The Crust:
1/2 c almonds
1/2 c walnuts
5–8 soaked and pitted dates
4 tbs shredded coconut, unsulfured and unsweetened (optional)
2 tsp vanilla (optional)
1 tsp cinnamon (optional)

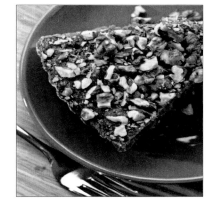

Tip: Soak almonds and walnuts in water or chai tea for a couple of hours. Drain and allow to air dry 1-2 hours. Toss nuts periodically to speed up drying.

Combine all ingredients. Spread mixture inside a glass pie pan.

The Topping (three different layers):
4 bananas cut into slices
4 tbs shredded, unsweetened, and dried coconut
1 c fresh strawberries or blueberries

Add sliced bananas, dried coconut, and, finally, the blueberries on top of the crust. Serve immediately, or refrigerate for later.

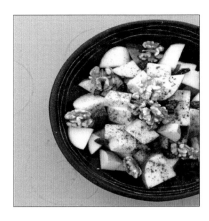

SUNRISE BREAKFAST
Serves 1–2

apple, cut in chunks (option: all varieties)
1/4 of a lemon, squeezed over apples
a sprinkle of sea salt
organic sweetener to taste (optional)
a few sprinkles of cinnamon
granola or sprouted, dehydrated, spiced buckwheat
raw pecans, almonds, or walnuts
organic raisins
dried apricots
pineapple
cherries

Mix all ingredients.

SPROUTED RAW BUCKWHEAT CEREAL
Serves 1–2

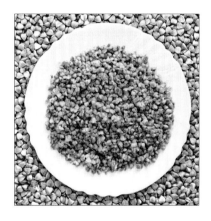

Soak 1 1/2 cups hulled buckwheat for about six hours.
Drain into a colander.
Let sprout in purified water for approximately two days.
(Be sure to pour off old water and refresh often.)
Add a few pours of agave nectar and sprinkle with 1/4 tsp cinnamon and a small pinch
of sea salt, cloves, and allspice.
Add nut milk and enjoy.
Or dehydrate at 118° Fahrenheit until dry, approximately six hours (optional).

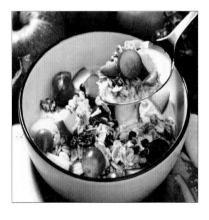

JACK SPRAT...APPLE JACK CEREAL
Serves 1–2
A lightly-spiced, sweet, and very dense crunchy breakfast cereal.

1 orange
1/4 c dried apples cut into small pieces (soak in liquid to soften texture)
1/2 c cashew pieces
2 tsp organic sweetener (optional)
1/4 tsp cinnamon
a dash of nutmeg
1/2 banana (optional)
a sprinkle of unsulfured and unsweetened coconut (optional)
1/4 c blueberries (optional)

Squeeze orange juice with pulp into cereal bowl. Add organic sweetener, cinnamon, and nutmeg. Stir, then mix in cashews and apples. Top with banana slices, grapes, raisins, or optional blueberries. Enjoy!

SNACKS

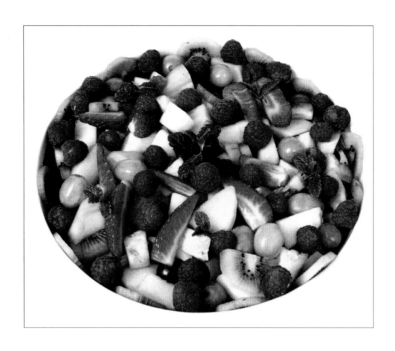

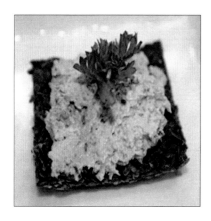

WALLY'S WALNUT PÂTÉ
Serves 1–2
We eat this all the time with sliced apples, romaine lettuce wraps, or stuffed celery. It's so easy to prepare and oh so delicious!

2 stalks celery
1 large red bell pepper (or 2–3 medium carrots)*
2 c walnuts
1 large scallion (green onion)
1/2–1 tsp sea salt
1/16–1/8 tsp cayenne pepper (optional)

The scallion can be substituted with 1/2–1 clove peeled garlic or chipotle may be used instead of cayenne pepper. If you need to make this in a hurry, you *can* substitute the large bell pepper for fire-roasted red bell peppers in olive oil or water.

Combine all ingredients in a food processor, placing walnuts on top, and blend until smooth or pulse-chop for more texture.

Versatility of Recipe:

Use as a dip, side dish, salad dressing, sandwich spread, or with apple slices, cucumber slices, stuffed zucchini, stuffed celery, romaine lettuce wrap, stuffed tomatoes (cherry, roma or regular), and stuffed red bell peppers on organic crackers.
Serving suggestions: Cut recipe in half for single servings.

* NOTE: Please contact your natural health care provider if you have insulin challenges.

CHICKY BABY CHICKEN SALAD
Serves 2–4

1/4 c sunflower seeds
1 c cashews
1 c pecans
1 cucumber (peeled, seeded, and cut into chunks)
2 green onions, cut into smaller pieces
1 celery stick, cut into smaller chunks
juice of 1/2 lemon
1 tsp dried dill
1/2 tsp sea salt
1/4 tsp curry powder (or to taste)
1/2 apple
1 avocado (optional—tastes great!)

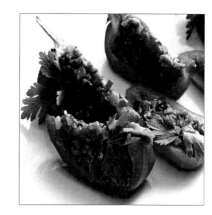

Put the nuts, seeds, seasonings, and lemon juice in food processor. Pulse for a few seconds until the pieces are smaller. Add remaining ingredients, including avocado. Pulse for a few more seconds until mixture is in smaller bits but not smooth. Spoon into red peppers or serve in a romaine wrap. You will love it!

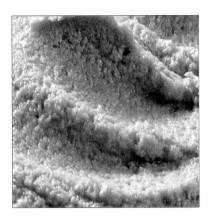

FRED AND GINGER'S ALMOND PÂTÉ*
Serves 1–2

2 tbs grated ginger
2 cloves garlic
1 tsp sea salt
2 c almonds
juice of 2 lemons (approximately 4 tbs) (Meyer lemons for less tart)
1/2 c filtered water, only as needed

Process ginger, garlic, and sea salt until well mixed. Add almonds and process while adding lemon juice. Add water *only* as needed for a hummus-like texture

*Enjoy with a *nori* roll, use as a lettuce wrap, or stuff tomatoes or red bell peppers.

ADAM AND EVE'S APPLESAUCE
Serves 2–4
Unlike cooked applesauce, this is a very fast, delicious, and easy recipe. You can use your food processor to pulse your own textures if you prefer a chunkier texture to a smoother one.

3 apples
2 tbs organic sweetener (optional)
1/2 tsp cinnamon
1/4 tsp vanilla

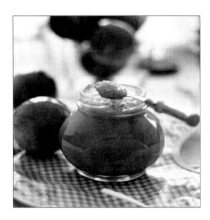

Slice apples into large chunks. No need to peel the apples! Place the apples and all other ingredients into your food processor and blend to your desired consistency.

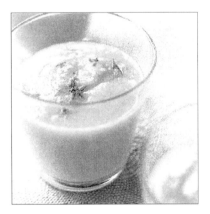

STRAWBERRY BANANAMANGO PUDDING
Serves 1–2

1 banana, peeled
1 mango, skinned and stoned
10 strawberries
2 dates, stoned (optional because this is a very sweet pudding)

Chop the dates. Put everything in a food processor and blend until it looks like a pudding.

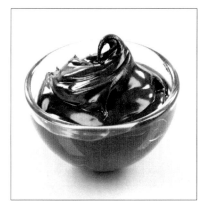

CAROB PUDDING

2 bananas
2 avocados
1/4 c carob powder

Put avocados, bananas, and carob powder into a food processor. Process until smooth. Layer into a parfait glass, and scoop some on top of strawberries or on fresh fruit. Sprinkle with unsweetened, unsulfured coconut (optional).

LADY BUGS

Fuji apples
raw almond butter
goji berries

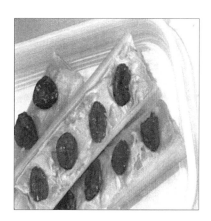

Slice the apples into thin rounds with a ceramic paring knife so that the apples don't oxidize and turn brown quickly. Another option is to soak them in diluted lemon water. Spread on the raw almond butter, and then sprinkle with a few handfuls of goji berries. Variations: Substitute celery for apples (lady bugs on a log) or large kale leaves (lady bugs on a leaf). Great for kids!

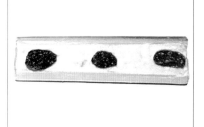

ANTS ON A LOG
Serves 1–2
Kids' favorite! And I love them myself as well!

stalks of celery
raw almond butter
raisins

Wash the celery stalks and trim the ends. Fill with raw almond butter. Cut into fourths. Top with raisin "ants."

CHOCOHOLICS

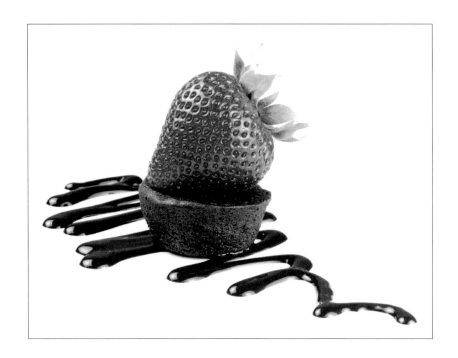

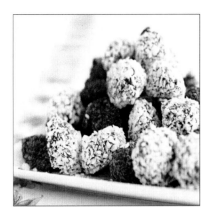

FREDDY'S FABULOUS FUDGE BALLS
Makes 12–24 Balls
These fudge balls are amazingly fudgy, rich enough to satisfy the most passionate chocoholics!

2 c dates, pitted and soaked
2 c almond butter
1/2 c organic carob powder
shredded coconut, unsulfured and unsweetened (optional)

In a food processor, blend the dates to a smooth paste. Add the remaining ingredients and process until smooth. Remove from the food processor and form into round balls, and then refrigerate.

Note: These will last for a long time if refrigerated!

BANANA CAROB TURTLES
Serves 1–2
A yummy, yummy, frozen banana treat that will remind you of Chocolate Turtles.

bananas
pecans
cinnamon
carob powder

Take ripe bananas and cut them into 3/4 pieces. Take 1/2 of a pecan and press lightly into the banana pieces. Top with a dash of cinnamon and carob. Freeze for one hour.

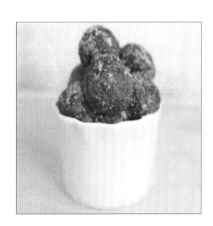

BLACK FOREST CAROB POUND CAKE WITH CAROB FUDGE FROSTING
Serves 2–4
This cake is really decadent and rich. Only sample a small piece to start.

Cake
1 3/4 c Brazil nuts
1 3/4 c cashews
1 tsp sea salt
3 c soaked and pitted dates
1 c carob powder
3 c shredded coconut, unsulfured and unsweetened

Frosting
1 c pitted and soaked dates
1/4 c carob powder
1/4 c grape seed oil or extra-virgin olive oil
1 c water, as needed

To make the cake, process Brazil nuts and sea salt into a powder in a food processor. Slowly add dates. Empty into large mixing bowl and add carob and coconut. Mix well and form into a cake shape. Shape cake by lining a container with parchment paper. Press into a container, fold over, and pull out. Peel off the parchment paper. Add frosting with spatula, then refrigerate to harden for at least one hour.

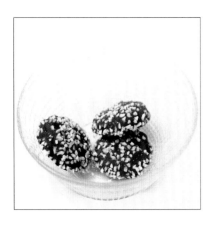

CRISPY CRUNCHY COOKIE
Makes 12–24 Cookies
Cookies that actually CRUNCH! YUMMMMMMMMMMMM!

1 c buckwheaties, buckwheat that has been soaked for six hours, thoroughly rinsed, drained and then dried in the dehydrator or air dry until crunchy.
1/2 c walnuts (or other nuts you like), we use soaked or dehydrated nuts to remove phytates and make them more digestible
6 Medjool dates
1/4 c water if needed, add a little at a time as needed
1 tbs almond butter or other nut butter
a pinch of sea salt, to taste
Other ingredients vary, depending on what flavor of cookies you want.

Process the buckwheaties in the food processor until mealy. Add the nuts and process briefly to chop them. Next, add the dates and process until doughy. Add a pinch of sea salt, if you want it. Then process briefly to distribute. Add a little water (or vanilla extract if you use it) if needed to make the dough hold together better. Then add the almond butter and finish processing the dough. Form into balls, squishing the dough together well so it will hold its shape and flatten into a cookie shape. Serve with nut milk or your favorite beverage! For more crunch, roll cookies in chopped nuts

You can leave these as is and have "Crunchy Nut Butter Cookies" or use one of the variations below or make up your own variation and let everyone know about it so we can try it, too!

Variations: "Chocolate Chip Cookies"—Process with some raw cacao nibs and raisins.
               "Raisin Spice Cookies"—Add some cinnamon, nutmeg, and ginger (or your favorite spices) and raisins.

SALADS

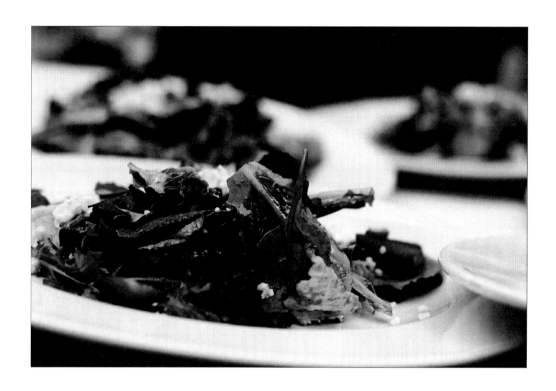

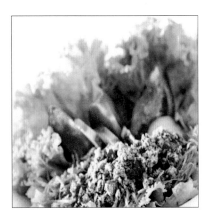

MOCK TUNA SALAD
Serves 4
A hearty sunflower pâté with diced celery, scallions, dried dill, and dulse flakes in a creamy, nut-based mayo.

The Salad
3 c soaked sunflower seeds, dried and ground
3–4 celery stalks, diced
1/2 bunch scallions, diced (green onions)
2 tbs dulse flakes
1/8–1/4 c dried dill (I prefer fresh diced dill)

The Dressing
1 1/2 c coconut water, unsweetened almond milk, or water
3–6 garlic cloves, peeled
1 c freshly squeezed lemon juice (preferably Meyer)
1 tbs sea salt
2 1/2 c raw cashews, pine nuts, macadamias, or a combination
1/2 c stone-ground mustard

In a large mixing bowl, combine all salad ingredients and toss to mix thoroughly. In a blender, combine all the dressing ingredients and blend well. Pour dressing over the salad, toss, and mix well.

Note: Soak sunflower seeds in pure water for two to four hours. Then drain and dry in dehydrator or air dry by mixing frequently to prevent mold.

MARINATED BROCCOLI WITH CRANBERRIES AND ALMONDS
Serves 4–6

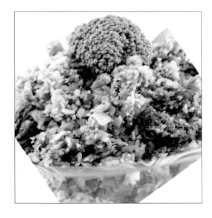

The Salad
4 c pulse-chopped broccoli florets (or left over additional veggies and fruits)*
1/2 c dried organic cranberries or blueberries
1/2 c slivered raw almonds

The Dressing
1/2 c apple or date juice or other fruit juice
1/4 c balsamic vinegar
1/2 c extra-virgin olive oil   1–3 cloves garlic, peeled
1/16 tsp cayenne pepper   4 sprays Bragg Liquid Aminos
1/4 c apple cider vinegar   1/2-3/4 tsp sea salt
organic sweetener to taste

In a large mixing bowl, combine chopped florets and toss in the bowl lightly. In a processor or blender, combine all dressing ingredients. Blend until smooth. Pour dressing over salad, mix well, and serve.

*Celery, cucumber, apples, scallions, raisins, carrots, zucchini, bell peppers, squash, and raw nuts all totaling four cups.

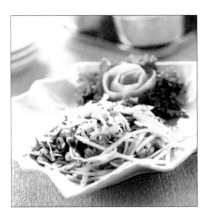

THAI ME TO THE MOON COLESLAW
Serves 3–4

The Salad
3 c finely-shredded green or napa cabbage
1 c peeled and shredded zucchini
1 c shredded carrot
1 bunch of fresh basil, mint, cilantro, with stems removed and leaves chopped
1/2 c raw, unsalted nuts
(Lightly drizzle a little extra-virgin olive oil and sea salt or Herbamare, and toss to mix.
You can use peanuts if you have no nut allergies.)

The Dressing
2 tbs fresh lemon juice
2 cloves garlic, peeled
2 tbs apple cider vinegar
1 one-inch piece ginger, peeled
1/4 c organic tamari or Bragg Liquid Aminos
1 tsp chili powder
1 1/2 tbs curry powder
organic sweetener to taste
1/4 c extra-virgin olive oil

In a large mixing bowl, combine all salad ingredients. Toss to mix thoroughly. In a processor or blender, combine all dressing ingredients. Blend until smooth. Pour dressing over salad, mix well. Sprinkle nuts over the top or prior to dressing and serve.

CAT SALAD (CORN, AVOCADO, TOMATO)
Serves 2–4

2 c fresh corn off the cob
1 avocado, cut into half-inch cubes
1 pint cherry tomatoes, halved
1/2 c finely diced red onion
1/2 red bell pepper (optional)

Dressing
2 tbs extra-virgin olive oil
1/2 tsp grated lime zest
1 tbs fresh lime juice
1/4 c chopped cilantro
1/4 tsp sea salt
1/4 tsp pepper

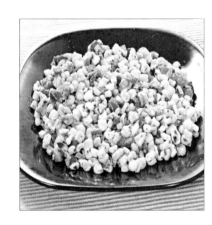

Combine the corn, avocado, tomatoes, and onion in a large glass bowl. Mix together the dressing ingredients in another bowl, pour over the salad, and gently toss to mix.

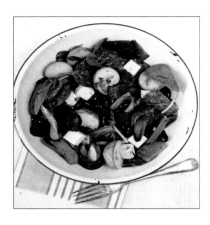

NAPA SPINACH SALAD
Serves 4–6
This quick, simple coleslaw is a real favorite. Make it as spicy as you like!

1 large head of napa cabbage (*wong bok*), medium sliced, lengthwise, coleslaw style
2 c roughly chopped fresh spinach
1/2 red bell pepper, julienned

<u>Dressing</u>
3 tbs lemon juice
3 tbs rice vinegar
2 tbs sesame oil
2 tbs extra-virgin olive oil
2 tsp red pepper flakes
sea salt and black pepper to taste

Combine all vegetables in a large bowl. Whisk dressing and ingredients in a small bowl, then pour over vegetables and toss.

<u>Note</u>: Optional items include tomato, cucumber, mushrooms, carrots, and radishes.

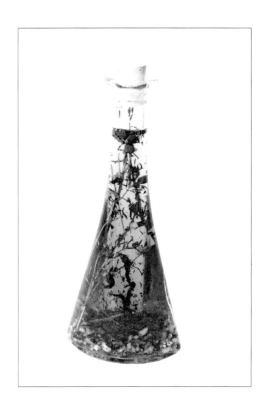

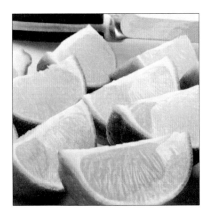

LIME VINAIGRETTE
Serves 1–2
This dressing tastes fabulous on fresh fruits and vegetable salads.

1/4 c fresh lime juice
organic sweetener to taste
1/2 tsp sea salt
1 clove garlic chopped
2 tsp finely-grated ginger
1/2 c extra-virgin olive oil

Pour the lime juice into a small bowl and whisk in the sugar and sea salt until dissolved. Add the garlic and ginger. Slowly add the olive oil in a steady stream, whisking constantly.

CHEF SHARYNNE'S BALSAMIC VINAIGRETTE HOUSE DRESSING
Serves 1–2

1/2 c lemon juice (or Meyer lemons)
1/4 c grape seed oil or extra-virgin olive oil
1/16–1/8 tsp cayenne pepper
1/4 c apple cider vinegar
1/8 c white (clear in color) or brown balsamic vinegar
1–3 peeled garlic cloves
1/4 tsp Bragg Liquid Aminos
1/2–3/4 tsp sea salt
1/4 c apple juice

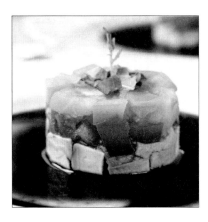

Mix all ingredients in a food processor. Blend until creamy.
Reblend if dressing separates while refrigerated.

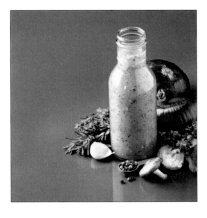

ITALIAN DRESSING
Serves 2–4
This one is jumping with herbs! The longer it sits, the better it tastes.

1 c extra-virgin olive oil
1 c fresh basil
1 c fresh parsley
1/2 c dried Italian seasoning
2 scallions (green onions)
2 tsp onion
1 lemon juiced
2 cloves peeled garlic
organic sweetener to taste
1/2 tsp sea salt

Blend all ingredients in a processor and chill for at least one hour.

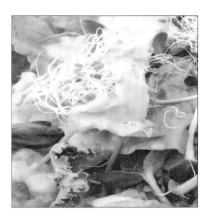

"Goddess in the Raw" Dressing
Serves 1–2
If you like garlic, you'll love this one!

2–3 limes
3/4 c apple cider vinegar
1 bunch scallions (green onions)
1/2 bunch parsley
4 cloves peeled garlic
1 tbs extra-virgin olive oil

Mix all ingredients by hand or in a food processor. Blend until well mixed.

Tahini Dressing
Serves 1–2
This dressing is a nice change from the oil that's in most dressings.

2 tbs tahini (similar to nut butters in consistency)
1/2 lemon, juiced
1/2 orange, juiced
1/2 c parsley
1/2–1 tsp organic sweetener to taste

Blend all ingredients in a processor or blender.

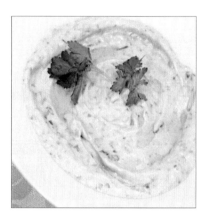

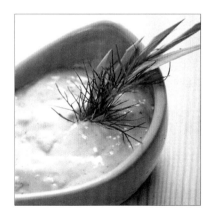

Dill Vinaigrette Dressing
Serves 1–2
This is a zippy vinaigrette infused with dill.

3 tbs extra-virgin olive oil
2 tbs apple cider vinegar
3 tbs dill
2 tbs parsley
1 clove peeled garlic
1/2 tsp sea salt
a pinch of black pepper

Blend all ingredients in a processor or blender.

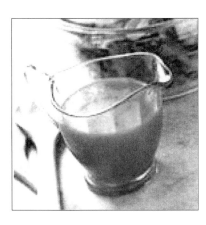

FRENCH DRESSING
Serves 1–2

1/4 c flax oil
2 tsp apple cider vinegar
1 clove peeled garlic
1/4 tsp ground yellow mustard seed
1/4 tsp paprika
1/4 tsp black pepper
1/2 tsp sea salt
organic sweetener to taste

Blend all ingredients in a processor or blender.

SOUPS

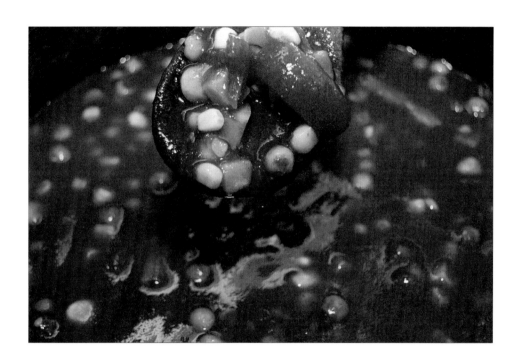

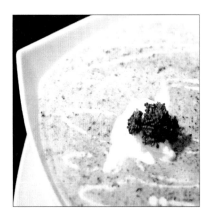

CREAM OF BROCCOLI SOUP
Serves 6–8
A powerful anti-cancer food; very smooth and creamy!

3 c water
1 c almonds*
organic sweetener to taste
2 c broccoli florets
1 avocado
1/2–1 peeled garlic clove
1 tbs extra-virgin olive oil
1 tsp onion
1 1/2 tsp sea salt
1/4 tsp cumin
1/4–3/4 tsp black pepper
1/16–1/8 tsp cayenne pepper (optional)

In a Vita-Mix or blender, combine water, almonds, and agave nectar until smooth. It can be warmed to 118° Fahrenheit, using the thermometer. Add the remaining ingredients and blend until smooth. Add additional sea salt to taste if needed.

* Note: For a creamier soup, soak almonds overnight if you have the time.

AVO-CUMBER SOUP
1 Serving
A wonderful end-of-summer soup, simple and refreshing, with a hint of dill!

1 avocado
1 cucumber
4 tbs dill weed
2 tsp freshly-squeezed lemon
1/2 tsp sea salt
1/16–1/8 tsp cayenne pepper (optional)
1/4 c corn (optional)
1 cherry tomato, sliced (optional)

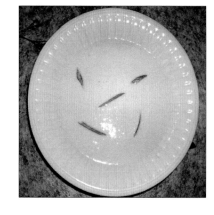

Combine all ingredients in a blender or Vita-Mix. Blend until smooth and creamy.

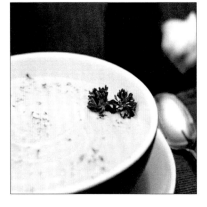

CREAMY BLG AVOCADO SOUP (BASIL, LIME, AND GINGER)
Serves 2–4

1 lime, juiced
3 c coconut water
1 one-inch peeled ginger
2 tsp chickpea *miso*
1/8–1/4 tsp cayenne or ground chili flakes (optional)
1 small handful of basil leaves
1 large avocado or 2 small

Blend all the soup ingredients together in a blender until completely smooth. Taste and adjust seasonings if necessary.

Suggested garnishes are chopped chives, cherry tomatoes, cucumbers, bell peppers, and seaweed.

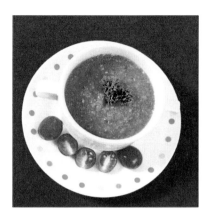

SPANISH GAZPACHO TRADITIONALE
Serves 2–4

10 medium ripe tomatoes
1/2 cucumber (about three-inch pieces)
1/2 red bell pepper
2 cloves garlic
2–3 tbs extra-virgin olive oil
1/8–1/4 tsp cayenne (optional)

Add all soup ingredients in the blender and blend until smooth.
Let soup sit in the refrigerator for a few hours before garnishing and serving.
Gazpacho is also better the next day.

<u>Suggested Garnishes</u>

2 tbs chopped green onion or chives
1/4 c chopped parsley
1/2 c sliced cherry tomatoes
1/2 c diced cucumbers
diced avocado
1–2 tbs ground flax or sesame seeds to be used as bread crumbs (optional)
a drizzle of extra-virgin olive oil (optional)

SPANISH GAZPACHO TRADITIONALE

LET'S GET SPROUTING 101

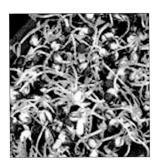 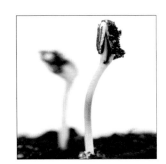 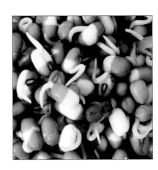

WHY DO WE "SPROUT"? NUTRITION

The tiny seeds are packed with stored nutrients just waiting for the moisture to start the germination process. Germination is simply the birth and growth of a baby plant, and it is both fascinating and wonderful, just like the birth of a child.

A common sunflower seed, for example, is only ¼-inch long, but it contains the blueprint necessary to provide for the development of a six-foot plant. A grain of wheat increases its vitamin E content 300% after only two days of growth and the B_2 vitamin Riboflavin jumps from 13 mg (milligrams) to 54 mg in the sprout. In general, B vitamins can increase 300% to 1,400%, depending on the variety.

Enzymes that start the chemical process of a developing plant are abundant in sprouts and help with digestion. Protein production in sprouts is quite dramatic since it is needed for the growth and development of cells.

Alfalfa sprouts contain 3.8% protein and sunflower sprouts contain 4.0%. This compares with Boston and Bibb lettuce, which contain 1.2%; New Zealand spinach, 2.6%'; and iceberg lettuce, with less than 1% protein. Minerals also increase during germination. The Potassium content of alfalfa sprouts is 870 mg (per 100 g) while Boston lettuce has 264 mg.

Alfalfa has 210 mg Calcium, and New Zealand spinach has 2.6 mg. The addition of liquid help to the soak and/or rinse water increases mineral content to levels that are as much or more than growing the plants in soil.

Sprouts are excellent food to feed your family, for very little money. A pound of alfalfa greens, for example, starts with only five tablespoons of seeds, costing about twenty-five cents.

Where else can you get organically grown greens for that price! Even if you do get organic produce, it often comes from far away. The costs of transporting food across continents or international borders are driven by politics, price of oil, and other factors we cannot control and which do not serve the farmer or the consumer. When you grow your own, you get the freshness factor.

Let's face it, a head of lettuce that is picked a week ago, transported across the country, and stored in a warehouse and on grocery shelves is not as vibrant as the one freshly picked from your garden. Sprouts are alive and grow right up to the time you put them on your plate.

The nutrients are in their prime and the enzymes are abundant. This "live food factor" delivers to us all of nature's secret ingredients that old produce no longer has to offer.

Is it organic? Of course! You can be sure because you are the grower. No questions about organic verification are necessary. Always buy organic sprouting seeds. If they don't sprout in the normal given time, you have a bad batch.

Keep your receipt after purchase and return to the store for credit. A harvest of home-grown indoor organic greens and beans is available year-round, whether you live in Hawaii or Alaska, in January or July.

The sprouts grow themselves. All you have to do is keep them warm and moist. New techniques such as using an automatic sprouting machine like the FreshLife Automatic Sprouter make sprouting fast and simple. There is no need to presoak or wash.

Germination occurs usually within twelve to sixteen hours, not days, if done manually. You can grow bushels of fresh young sprouts in little space and little time. Green thumb not required!

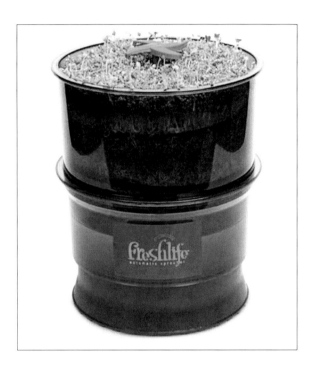

FRESHLIFE AUTOMATIC SPROUTER®

This sprouting method can be used with a variety of different seeds, grains, and beans. With soybeans and chickpeas, rinse four times a day and make sure they are well drained or they'll rot. The following is a timetable for manual sprouting with the desired length of each type of sprout and how long it should take.

SPROUTING TIMETABLE

Bean, Grain, or Seed	Sprout Length	Days to Sprout
alfalfa	1"	3 - 5
barley	1/8"	3 - 5
chickpeas	3/4 - 1"	5 - 8
millet	1/8"	3 - 5
mung bean	1/2 - 1 1/2"	3 - 6
pumpkin	opened seed	3 - 5
radish	1/2 - 1"	2 - 4
rice	1/8"	3 - 4
sesame	opened seed	2 - 3
soybean	3/4 - 1"	4 - 6
sunflower	opened seed	5 - 8
wheat	1/8"	2 - 4

SPROUT SEEDS

Sprouting grains, beans, almonds, and other seeds is a much-overlooked way to use these basic foods. You'll find ways to use sprouts in various recipes in this section. You may also use them in place of green leaves in the winter. As a sandwich filling, sprouts give body and flavor. The table below will show how simple it is to prepare sprouts. Use dry beans, whole hulled sunflower and similar seeds, and shelled, unblanched almonds.

Soak seeds in water overnight in a Mason jar. Next morning, drain off the water and rinse the seeds until the water runs clear. Drain well.

Place screening or cheesecloth over the jar opening and attach it with the metal ring or use a rubber band to hold the seeds in. A nylon or stainless steel screen may be purchased at your local home improvement store. Large seeds may be grown and rinsed in a colander.

Set the jar on its side and rinse the seeds two to three times a day for one to four days. Refrigerate the sprouts when they are ready.

Variety	Number of days	Amount of seeds	Serving suggestions	Health benefits
alfalfa	3–4	1½ tablespoon	raw in salads and sandwiches, or chopped in baked goods	vitamin C, carotene, chlorophyll, vitamin K, and many other nutrients
almonds	1	1 cup raw or roasted	snacks, salads, hors d'oeuvres	lower blood cholesterol level, reduce heart disease, rich in vitamin E, and useful source of calcium
adzuki beans (or azuki beans)	2–3	1 cup	sprout and use in salad, chili or wraps	favorable calcium to phosphorous ratio (4:1) for helping in preventing osteoporosis
black beans (Black turtle bean)	1–3	1 cup	sprout and use in salad, chili, or wraps; use in bean soup	beneficial to kidneys and reproductive function and diuretic effect; black bean juice is effective for hoarseness, laryngitis, kidney stones, bed-wetting, urinary difficulty, and hot flashes due to menopause
garbanzo beans (chickpea)	1–2	1 cup	sprout and use to make hummus or toss in salad or soup	beneficial to pancreas, stomach, and heart; contains more iron than other legumes and is also a good source of unsaturated fats
lentils	1–3	1 cup	sprout for soup and lentil salad	for diuretic effect, beneficial to the heart and circulation, stimulates the adrenal system, and increases vitality of the kidney
mung beans (the common Chinese sprouts)	2–3	1 cup	in Chinese recipes: salads, in a miso soup, and as stir-fried vegetable	detoxifies the body and beneficial to the liver and gall bladder and diuretic effect
soybeans	2–4	1 cup	sprout, add to salads, or mash for sandwich spread	helps lower risk of heart disease, eases constipation, improves intestinal health, steadies blood sugar level, eases menopausal symptoms, may reduce the risk of breast cancer, and rich in iron, calcium, and potassium
sunflower seed	1–2	1 cup	use in pâtés, raw snacks, tabbouleh, fruit salads	provides good levels of vitamin E and B and iron; contains linoleic acid that lowers blood cholesterol levels and prevents heart diseases

Nutrients

Legumes are not only high in protein but also in fat and carbohydrate. They are rich sources of Potassium, Calcium, Iron, and several B vitamins.

Juice's preparation and dosage

Simmer one cup of beans in five cups of water for an hour (remove the juice and continue cooking the bean). Take half a cup of juice a half hour before meals as a remedy for nephritis and most other kidney complaints. Regular drinking of the juice with meals increases mothers' milk. (Source: *Eat Your Way to Better Health* by Dr. Gene Spiller).

Soaking Legumes

Soak legumes for twelve hours or overnight in four parts water to one part legume. For best results, change the water once or twice. Lentils and whole-dried peas require shorter soaking while soybeans and garbanzos need to soak longer. Soaking also promotes and improves digestibility because the gas-causing enzyme inhibitors and tri-saccharides in legumes are released into the soak water. Be sure to discard the soak water.

Grain and Seed Milks

Seed Milk
1/2 cup seed (pumpkin, sesame, or sunflower)
1 cup warm water
a dash of kelp or sea salt

Soak seeds overnight. Drain and throw away soak water. Blend with warm water and kelp or sea salt. Use as is, or strain and use pulp in breads, cookies, etc.

Almond Milk
1/4 cup almonds (walnuts or other nuts may be substitutes)
2 cups warm water
a dash of kelp or sea salt

Follow recipe of seed milk.
Option: remove skins after soaking almonds, especially for persons with digestion challenges

Almond Milk Shake
Replace water with warm fruit juice in almond milk recipe, or add fruit, 2 tablespoons grain coffee or 1/4 cup carob powder. Blend all ingredients together.

Sprout Grain Milk
1 cup grain (oats, rice millet, or barley)
2 cups water
Sprout grain for 3 days (refer to how to sprout seeds)
Blend with water and strain. Use pulp for bread, soups, etc.

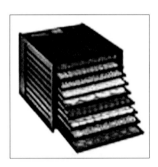

FOOD DEHYDRATION: AN ALTERNATE METHOD OF FOOD PRESERVATION

Dehydration is another method of preserving food by removing most of its water content. Dehydrated foods are lighter in weight, easier to store, and easier to pack and bring along than canned goods or frozen goods. If properly packaged, dehydrated food will last indefinitely. Archeologists have found dehydrated foods in the tombs of the pharaohs that still had nutritional value although it was centuries old.

The trick to proper preservation of dehydrated goods is to remove enough moisture, keep oxygen out, and keep away from as much light as possible. Most fruits need 80% of water removed. Most vegetables need 95% of water removed. Dehydrated meat needs to be dried to between leathery to brittle. Consistent dehydration is easier if produce is sliced thin and slices are all fairly consistent in size. The light does not hurt the quality of the food but can cause dehydrated food to lose its color (same as with canned goods). Vacuum sealing is a good way to remove air from packaged dehydrated goods. They can also be packed in zip-locked bags or dry canning jars.

DEHYDRATION FORMULA FOR FRESH WEIGHT VERSUS DRIED WEIGHT

After peeling, coring, etc., weigh prepared produce. (For example, peeled, cored, sliced apples weigh 10 lbs [pounds].) See water content of fruits or vegetables (apples = 84%).

The total weight of the water equals the weight of prepared fruit/vegetable multiplied by the percent of water content (10 × 0.84 = 8.4 pounds of water). Most fruits need 80% of water removed. Most vegetables need 95% of water removed. Multiply the total weight of water by the percent of water to be removed. (For apples: 8.4 × 0.80 = 6.72 lbs of water to remove.)

To find out how much the produce should weigh after dehydrating, subtract the weight of water to be removed from the weight of the fresh product. (For apples, 10 lbs prepared apples minus 6.72 lbs of water = 3.28 lbs of dried apples. In this technique, the apples would be sufficiently dehydrated when they weigh about 3¼ lbs.)

FRUITS AND VEGETABLES' WATER CONTENT

Apples...85%
Apricots...85%
Bananas..76%
Bean sprouts...92%
Broccoli...91%
Cabbage, raw...92%
Cantaloupe..91%

Carrots, raw...88%
Cauliflower, raw...91%
Celery...94%
Cherries, raw...80%
Coconut, dried..7%
Collards, boiled..91%
Corn, sweet or fresh.......................................74%
Cucumbers, raw...96%
Eggplant, raw..92%
Grapefruit, raw..88%
Grapes..82%
Kale..87%
Lettuce head...96%
Okra, boiled...91%
Olives..80%
Onions..89%
Oranges...86%
Papayas, raw...89%
Parsley, raw...86%
Peaches, raw...90%
Pears, raw...82%
Peas, raw..81%
Peppers, green...94%

The secret to successful dehydration of crackers, breads, and cookies is thickness. Make sure the thickness does not exceed 1/8 - 1/4" thickness unless the recipe calls for it to be thicker. Any increased thickness will require longer dehydrating time and increased temperature not to exceed 118°.

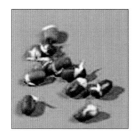

Adzuki Beans: A very nutritious maroon-colored legume used as a sprouted seed. Adzuki beans are high in Vitamins A, B, C, E, Calcium, Iron, Niacin. Adzuki contains all the essential amino acids except Tryptophan and is loaded with flavor and 25% protein.

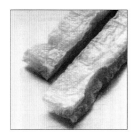

Agar: A natural thickening and jelling agent derived from seaweed.

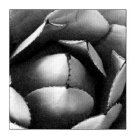
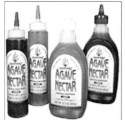

Agave: A natural sweetener made from the juice of the agave cactus plant. The cactus is also used to make Tequila and has a lower glycemic index than honey, maple syrup or cane sugar. Available in light for a mild sweet flavor or dark for a mild molasses flavor. After further research this is **NOT** a healthy sweetener. It will elevate triglycerides and uric acid levels.

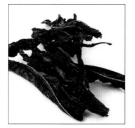

Alaria: a.k.a. Wakame a highly nutritious seaweed that adds a wonderful flavor to foods when the fish flavor needs to be emulated in a recipe.

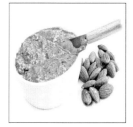

Almond Butter (raw): A creamy, thick spread made from ground raw almonds. It can be used to replace peanut butter when peanut allergies exist. Peanut butter, although organic is made from roasted nuts. This is a convenient pantry staple that can be used for quick recipes.

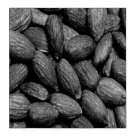

Almonds (raw/shelled): Raw nuts rich in Vitamins A, B, C, E, Calcium, Iron, Magnesium, Niacin, Phosphorus, Potassium, All Essential Amino Acids, and 20-25% Protein. This is a convenient pantry staple that can be used for quick recipes.

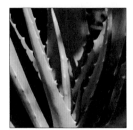

Aloe Vera: The juice from the leaves date back to centuries ago for soothing and healing of the skin. When buying, always buy the whole leaf and preservative-free.

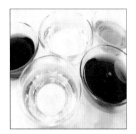

Apple Cider Vinegar (raw): A fruity vinegar made from apple juice. Always buy raw and un-pasteurized. This vinegar contains lots of healthy bacteria and enzymes for digestion.

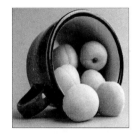

Apricots (dried): Always buy *un-sulfured* and keep in the refrigerator or freeze them for an extended shelf-life. Apricots are healthy because they contain lots of Beta carotene, the plant form of Vitamin A, which is a good anti-oxidant. They are also high in fiber and low in calories, and make a good snack. Ounce for ounce, dried apricots are an even healthier option as the drying process increases the concentration of the Beta carotene, fiber and also the levels of Potassium and Iron.

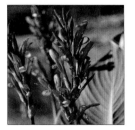

Arrowroot Powder: Arrowroot is an easily digested starch extracted from the roots of the arrowroot plant. The starch is used as a thickening agent in many foods such as puddings and sauces, and is also used in cookies and other baked goods. Arrowroot is extremely bland, making it suitable for neutral diets, especially for people who are feeling nauseous. It is not terribly nutritious, but some people believe that it helps to soothe upset stomachs, which is why many health food stores carry arrowroot cookies.

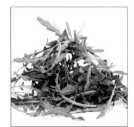

Arugula: a.k.a. "Rocket" A salad green with a peppery and slightly bitter flavor.

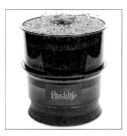

Automatic Sprouter: An appliance used to grow green leafy sprouts and wheatgrass. It's use requires no daily rinsing or draining. I highly recommend the Tribest FreshLife Automatic Sprouter.

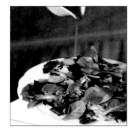

Balsamic Vinegar: An Italian vinegar made from grape juice with a distinct sweet and sour flavor. True balsamic vinegar (Aceto Balsamic Tradizionale) is aged a minimum of 10 years in wooden vats. The finer and most expensive is aged from 25-50 years.

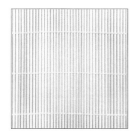

Bamboo Sushi Mat: Made of bamboo, this woven mat is essential for making Nori rolls.

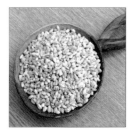

Barley (hulled): Hullless barley is intended for sprouting and contain loads of Vitamins A, B, C, E, Calcium, Iron, Magnesium, Niacin, Phosphorus, Potassium, Amino Acids and 15% Protein.

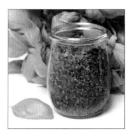

Basil: An important plant in Mediterranean and French cuisine. Brewed as a tea, basil is great for the gastrointestinal tract. It can relieve gas and even combat dysentery. Just like mint, the basil's closest relative, it is easy to cultivate in a garden or in a pot at home. And, of course, it has a pleasant and unique taste, which makes it an indispensable ingredient for the preparation of many tomato, fish and meat dishes.

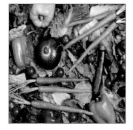

Beta-carotene: A nutrient found in red, green and orange vegetables that the body converts into Vitamin A.

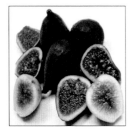

Black Mission Figs: A purple-black fig with a deep flavor and rich in Iron.

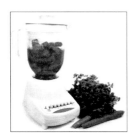

Blender: An electric kitchen appliance that purees and liquefies. The powerful high-speed types would be the Vita-Mix or K-Tec. I highly recommend the Vita-Mix. They've been around for over 80 years. Product features 7 or 10 year warranty directly from Vita-Mix. ChefSharynne.com is an affiliate provider.

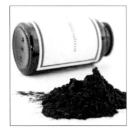

Blue-Green Algae: An excellent source of Protein, Chlorophyll, Beta-carotene, and many trace minerals. There are 3 types Klamath Lake, Spirulina and Chlorella. E-3 Live from Klamath Lake is highly recommended.

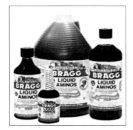

Bragg Liquid Aminos: A liquid seasoning made from soybeans and distilled water. Saltier than Nama Shoyu or Organic Tamari, however less expensive. Dilute when using so it won't over-power your recipe *(wheat-free)*.

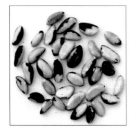

Brazil Nuts: Rich and creamy nuts an excellent source of Selenium. Their antioxidant properties help prevent cellular damage from free radicals. Free radicals are natural by-products of oxygen metabolism that may contribute to the development of chronic diseases such as cancer and heart disease.

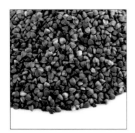

Buckwheat (unhulled): a.k.a. "buckwheat lettuce." Used for soil-grown sprouted greens. Buckwheat contains Rutrin, a medicinal chemical that strengthens capillary walls, reducing hemorrhaging in people with high blood pressure. Buckwheat contains D-chiro-inositol a component found to be deficient in Type II diabetes and Polycystic Ovary Syndrome. It is being studied for use in treating Type II diabetes. Buckwheat protein has been found to bind cholesterol tightly. It is being studied for reducing plasma cholesterol in people with an excess of this compound.

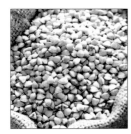

Buckwheat (raw/hulled): a.k.a. "groats". Buckwheat usually is sprouted, and used for cereal and dough. When the buckwheat is toasted it's called "Kashi".

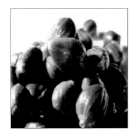

Capers: An unopened green flower buds of the *Capparis spinosa* (Capparidaceae - caper family - closely related to the cabbage family), a wild and cultivated bush that is grown mainly in Mediterranean countries (southern France, Italy, and Algeria) and also in California. Picked manually in the morning for the right size, sun-dried, then pickled in vinegar brine.

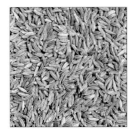

Caraway Seeds: Actually the fruit of a biennial herb in the parsley family. The seed is about 1/5 inch long and tapered at the ends. The hard seed shells have five pale ridges. These seeds will quickly lose their flavor. Store them in the refrigerator or freezer for a longer shelf-life.

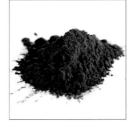

Carob Powder: a.k.a. "St. John's Fruit". A dark brown powder made from ground up carob seeds and the pods. This powder tastes similar to cocoa powder, but without the caffeine and is sweet to the taste. Buy preferably raw, however toasted will work. Sometimes the raw carob powder is difficult to find and quite pricey.

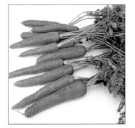

Carrots: Great for juicing. Carrots are high in Vitamins A, K, C, B6, B1 (thiamin), B3 (niacin), Dietary Fiber, Potassium, Manganese, Molybdenum, Phosphorus, Magnesium and Folate. *CAUTION:* For those individuals who must carefully monitor their insulin levels, beware of the high sugar content.

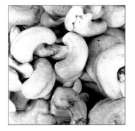

Cashews: They are sweet and make excellent creamy and smooth dressings and toppings. Cashews are rich in Copper, Magnesium, Tryptophan and Phosphorus. They are not considered raw so use them occasionally.

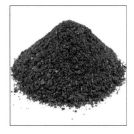

Cayenne Pepper: A powerful, pungent, stimulating taste and smelling pepper made by grinding dried pods of small chili peppers. Cayenne pepper is very beneficial for increasing circulation. Cayenne has also been used medicinally for thousands of years. Cayenne is often referred to as "chili", which is the Aztec name for cayenne pepper.

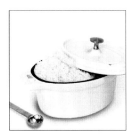

Celtic Sea Salt®Brand: Clean, unrefined, and hand-harvested natural Celtic Sea Salt, used in the proper manner, has reversed many a "chronic illness" and restored wholeness in just a few days. Because of its complex beneficial minerals and bio-electronic power it offers countless health benefits: it balances alkalinity/acidity levels, restores good digestion, and relieves allergies and skin diseases. The daily use of these natural salts along with a whole-grain-based diet could greatly reduce toxins and prevent ill-health. Loaded with over 80 minerals! Celtic sea salt may be safe for most hypertensive patients. Check with your medical practitioner first before using. ChefSharynne.com is an affiliate provider.

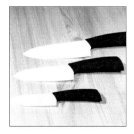

Ceramic Knives: Kyocera ceramic knives are great for cutting fruits, lettuce because they don't cause oxidation when they come in contact with the produce, which causes the brown discoloration. These do tend to be pricey. Need to be professionally sharpened.

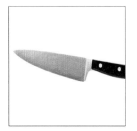

Chef's Knife: 7-10" knife with a broad blade. Used for slicing, chopping, dicing and mincing. Usually a 7-8" knife will work for most kitchen tasks. The Asian knife version is called a "Santoku". Some names to look for are Henckels, Global, Cutco and Kyocera.

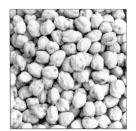

Chickpeas: a.k.a. "garbanzo or ceci beans" Chickpeas are great for sprouting and are a source of Zinc, Folate and Protein. They are very high in dietary fiber and a healthy source of carbohydrates for diabetics.

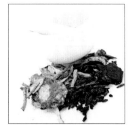

Chinese 5-spice Powder: An aromatic blend of cinnamon, cloves, fennel, star anise, and Szechwan peppercorns. Has a distinct "Asian" flavor.

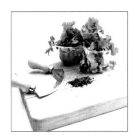

Cilantro: a.k.a. "Chinese Parsley" Cilantro is the leaf of the young coriander plant. It's a herb in the parsley family, similar to anise.

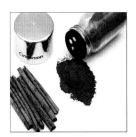

Cinnamon: There has been a lot of talk these days about cinnamon. According to some studies, cinnamon may improve blood glucose and cholesterol levels in people with Type 2 diabetes. The results of a study from 2003 in Pakistan showed lower levels of fasting glucose, triglycerides, LDL cholesterol and total cholesterol after 40 days with levels continuing to drop for 20 days after that.

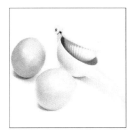

Citrus Press: This appliance will crush the inside of halved citrus fruits, thus releasing the juice. There are different sizes available for lemons, oranges and limes. This appliance is a MUST!

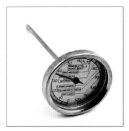

Cooking Thermometer: This appliance is used with your Vita-Mix processor when you don't want to exceed critical temperature of 112°-118° Fahrenheit. Temperatures above this range begin to destroy vital nutrients and enzymes.

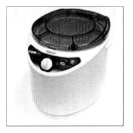

CuisineClean™: A kitchen appliance that kills 99.9% of a multitude of bacteria, pesticides, fungicides, dirt, sand without utilizing chemicals. It uses O3 (ozone) which is produced by an ozone generator. The same process that is used by Mother Nature after a storm and the air smells so refreshing. ChefSharynne.com is an affiliate provider.

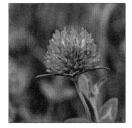

Clover Seeds: A small legume, great for sprouting. Rich in Vitamins A, B, C, E, K, Calcium, Iron, Magnesium, Phosphorus, Potassium, Zinc, Carotene, Chlorophyll, Amino Acids, Trace Elements, 35% Protein and excellent for Women.

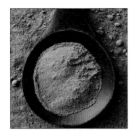

Cocoa Power (unsweetened): The process begins with the highest quality organic raw cacao beans and cold pressing them to make a dark brown paste called chocolate liquor. The paste or often called liquor is cold pressed at 112° Fahrenheit (sometimes even lower) to separate out its fat (cacao butter). What remains is a "cake" (also known as cocoa solids) this part is then cold milled to become organic, truly raw unsweetened cocoa powder.

This has the highest level of cocoa flavonols (improves cardiovascular health) because it's the least processed. Also, because the fat has been removed and it contains no extra ingredients such as sugar, it's the healthiest form of chocolate you can ever eat.

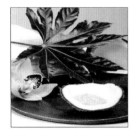

Coconut Oil: May have antioxidant properties, since the oil doesn't turn rancid and since it reduces our need for vitamin E, whereas unsaturated oils deplete vitamin E. The cholesterol-lowering properties of coconut oil are a direct result of its ability to stimulate thyroid function. In the presence of adequate thyroid hormone, cholesterol (specifically LDL-cholesterol) is converted by enzymatic processes to the vitally necessary anti-aging steroids, progesterone and DHEA. These substances are required to help prevent heart disease, senility, obesity, cancer and other diseases associated with aging and chronic degenerative diseases.

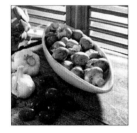

Cremini Mushrooms: These are closely related to common white mushrooms, but they're a bit more flavorful. The portabello mushroom is the fully matured cremini mushroom.

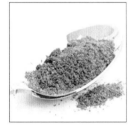

Cumin: A strong and pungent flavored spice that aids in digestion. Buy it whole or grind in a coffee grinder yourself.

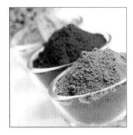

Curry Powder: Curry powder is a blend of up to 20 different herbs and spices, including the commonly used: cardamom, chiles, cinnamon, cloves, coriander, cumin, fennel, fenugreek, mace, nutmeg, pepper, poppy seeds, sesame seeds, saffron, tamarind and tumeric (which gives curry its characteristic golden color). In Indian cooking curry is freshly ground each day (making it far more flavorful and pungent than the mixes sold in the store). Curry quickly loses its pungency. It will keep for 2 months in an airtight container.

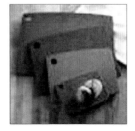

Cutting Board: A flat surface board used for cutting fruits and vegetables. The Epicurean unlike wood or bamboo cutting boards are designed to be dishwasher safe. They are knife friendly, maintenance-free and eco-friendly. All boards are made with eco-select paper from trees harvested under the guidelines of the North America Sustainable Forestry Standards. Sixty percent of the energy used to produce the raw material is from a renewable source. I highly recommend the Epicurean cutting board.

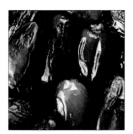

Dates: Three best varieties for Raw and Living food preparation: Medjool, Khadrawl and Honey. You can use dates pieces for a more economical option when the recipe calls for whole dates.

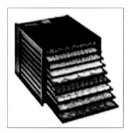

Dehydrator: A kitchen appliance for drying food indoor like fruits, vegetable, nuts, seed, fruit leathers, raw breads, crackers, cookies and bars. I personally recommend the Excalibur™, with corresponding Teflex or Paraflex sheets. These sheets will aid you in drying wet mixtures like fruit leathers and cracker batters. ChefSharynne.com is an affiliate provider.

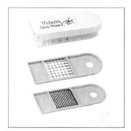

Dice: To cut food into very small cubes, usually ¼". This can be accomplished using a Vidalia Chop Wizard found at your local discount store. This appliance is another MUST!

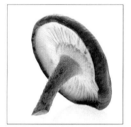

Dried Shiitake Mushrooms: Have a wonderful smoky flavor and a meaty texture. They are one of the most versatile mushrooms for their economical price. Shiitake mushrooms are the best all around dried mushrooms. Simply soak in purified water for 30 minutes to reconstitute them.

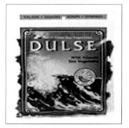

Dulse: A reddish-purple sea vegetable that can be ground into a powder and used as a salty condiment. Dulse contains Calcium, Potassium, Magnesium, Iron, Iodine, Manganese, Copper, Chromium, Zinc, and Vitamins A, B1, B2, B3, B6, B12, C and E.

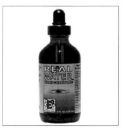

E2 Real Water: Did you know that most of the water you drink every day may actually be damaging your health. And it's not just plain water, how about juice, tea, coffee, soda? You see, nearly everything we drink has water as its foundation.

And, this also includes you! Your body is over 70% water. So doesn't it make sense, that you drink water and use water based products that help improve your health instead of harm it? Of course it does. E2 Real Water is also available through Silver Springs Water, a home delivery service in Las Vegas. Silver Springs is currently looking to expand its market share. For more details go to www.silverspringswaterlasvegas.com. E2 Real Water can be purchased at the retail level at most major health food chains and grocers.

Enzymes: Enzymes are made from amino acids, and they are proteins. Raw and Living Food is loaded with readily available enzymes and are easily absorbed by the body Enzymes are used by our cells to replenish our depleted cells.

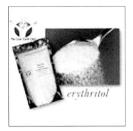

Erythritol: Erythritol™ occurs naturally in some fruits and fermented foods. As a sweetener, it is made from corn via a natural fermentation process. The properties of this great-tasting, natural sweetener are remarkable.   Erythritol is 80% as sweet as sugar. However, unlike sugar, which is high in calories, erythritol is almost calorie-free (4 calories). It scores just over zero on the glycemic index. That means it is totally safe for the insulin challenged and won't affect insulin levels. It is granulated, just like sugar, so it can be easily substituted for sugar in recipes. It is easy to digest - which means no gastrointestinal disturbance. Check with your medical practitioner first before using. Erythritol, when compared with other sugar alcohols, is also much more difficult for intestinal bacteria to digest, so it is unlikely to cause gas or bloating, unlike maltitol, sorbitol, or lactitol. Allergic side effects can be itching with hives.

Essential Fatty Acids (EFA's): Critical for energy, mental state, healthy skin and hair. Our bodies can't produce them and must get them from our food. Rich sources are seed oils, flax seeeds, pumpkin seeds and fish oils. Refined oils, heated oils, hydrogenated oils and saturated fats contain no EFA's.

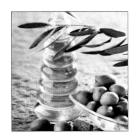

Extra-Virgin Olive Oil: Olive oil vendors choose the wording on their labels very carefully. EVOO should be stored in dark glass and out of the light to prevent oxidation and going rancid.

> **"100% Pure Olive Oil"** is often the lowest quality available in a retail store: better grades would have "virgin" on the label.

> **"Made from refined olive oils"** means that the taste and acidity were chemically controlled.

> **"Light olive oil"** means refined olive oil, with less flavor. All olive oil has 120 calories per tablespoon.

> **"From hand-picked olives"** implies that the oil is of better quality, since producers harvesting olives by mechanical methods are inclined to leave olives to over-ripen in order to increase yield.

> **"First cold press"** means that the oil in bottles with this label is the first oil that came from the first press of the olives. The word *cold* is important because if heat is used, the olive oil's chemistry is changed. It should be noted that extra-virgin olive oil is cold pressed, but not necessarily the first oils.

The label may indicate that the oil was bottled or packed in a stated country. This does not necessarily mean that the oil was produced there. The origin of the oil may sometimes be marked elsewhere on the label; it may be a mixture of oils from several places.

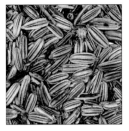

Fennel Seeds: Seeds that have a licorice-like flavor. Helps aid in digestion.

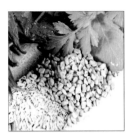

Fenugreek Seeds: A small legume used in sprouting and contains Vitamins A, B, C, E, Calcium, Iron, Magnesium, Phosphorus, Potassium, Zinc, Carotene, Chlorophyll, Phyto-nutrients and excellent for a woman's breast health, Amino Acids, trace elements, digestive aid, 30% Protein.

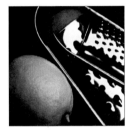

File Grater: Great for grating ginger, nutmeg and chocolate.

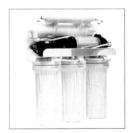

Filtered Water: Water is filtered through a carbon block. The carbon removes chlorine, some chemicals, heavy metals like lead and mercury.

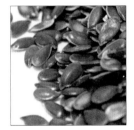

Flax Seeds: a.k.a. "linseed oil" Flax seeds contain high levels of lignans and Omega-3 fatty acids. Lignans are beneficial to the heart, contain anti-cancer properties. Studies performed on mice found reduced growth in specific types of tumors. (breast and prostate cancer) Flax may also lessen the severity of diabetes by stabilizing blood-sugar levels. Flax seeds may be used as a laxative due to the fiber content. Consuming large amounts of flax seed can impair the effectiveness of certain oral medications, due to its fiber content. In Raw and Living Food they are used as a thickener. They can be ground up and placed in beverages and sprinkled on salads. Flax seed contains Vitamins A, B, C, E, Calcium, Iron, Magnesium, Niacin, Phosphorus, Potassium, All Essential Amino Acids, Antioxidants, and approximately 20-25% Protein. Nutritional value is the same for all colors except yellow flax called Linola or Solin, which has a completely different oil profile and is very low in Omega-3 fatty acids.

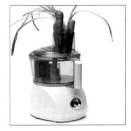

Food Processor: A kitchen appliance with interchangeable blades and cutting disks. Used for chopping, grinding, pureeing, slicing, and shredding. Most can be purchased for under $100. For more bang for your buck, the Hamilton Beach™ is an excellent value with a 14 cup capacity.

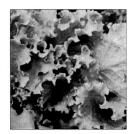

Frisée: A mild and bitter salad green with a feathery texture. Used commonly with mesclun mix. If you can't find in your grocery store you can substitute curly endive.

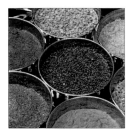

Garam Masala: "Garam" is an Indian word that means "warm" and "sala" means mix. Used as an exotic flavor with warmth. Contains: 4 whole cloves, 8 black peppercorns, Seeds from 2 green cardamom pods, ¼ tsp cinnamon, ¼ tsp nutmeg, A few strands of saffron.

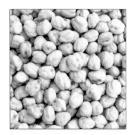

Garbanzo Beans: a.k.a. "chickpeas" have a delicious nutlike taste and buttery texture. They provide a good source of protein. A very versatile legume, they are a noted ingredient in many Middle Eastern and Indian dishes such as hummus, falafels and curries. While many people think of garbanzos as being beige in color, there are varieties that feature black, green, red and brown beans.

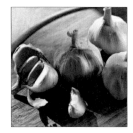

Garlic: Has many health benefits in preventing atherosclerosis (heart disease), high cholesterol, high blood pressure, and cancer.

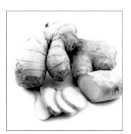

Ginger: The medical form of ginger a.k.a."Jamaica ginger". Used for digestive ailments, blood thinning and cholesterol lowering properties. CAUTION: Do not eat ginger if you are suffering from gallstones or are taking warfarin (a blood thinner). Ginger may decrease the joint pain from arthritis. Raw and Living food recipes use lots of ginger so use with caution if any of the above pertain to you. Ginger compounds can also control diarrhea with is the leading cause of infant death in developing countries. Ginger is also effective in treating nausea, sea sickness, morning sickness and chemotherapy.

Glycemic Index: A system that ranks foods according to how much and how quickly they raise blood sugar levels. The lower the index number the better and slower blood glucose levels will rise. There are many new organic products that are not chemical in nature. These can be used by diabetics rather than the artificial sweeteners on the market today. (NutraSweet, Sweet 'n Low, Somer Sweet, Equal, the pink stuff, the blue stuff, the yellow stuff) all contain aspartame which has been linked to CNS (central nervous system) disorders like Alzheimer's, dementia and brain tumors.

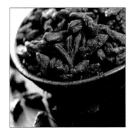

Goji Berries: Goji berries have been used for 6,000 years by herbalists in China, Tibet and India to:

· protect the liver
· help eyesight
· improve sexual function and fertility
· strengthen the legs
· boost immune function
· improve circulation
· promote longevity

Goji berries are rich in antioxidants, particularly carotenoids such as Beta-carotene and Zeaxanthin. One of Zeaxanthin's key roles is to protect the retina of the eye by absorbing blue light and acting as an antioxidant. In fact, increased intake of foods containing Zeaxanthin may decrease the risk of developing age-related macular degeneration (AMD), the leading cause of vision loss and blindness in people over the age of 65. Las Vegas casino mogul, Steve Wynn has AMD.

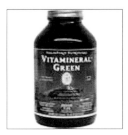

Green Powders: These are whole-food supplements that are made from dehydrated barley grasses, dehydrated wheat, blue-green algae and dehydrated green leafy vegetables.

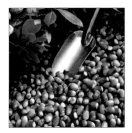

Hazelnuts: a.k.a. "filberts" Did you know they are one of the most nutritious nuts? Hazelnuts are a rich source of dietary fiber, Vitamin E, Magnesium, and heart healthy B vitamins. They reduce the risk of cardiovascular disease. Not only are hazelnuts a high-quality source of protein and fiber, they also contain a variety of antioxidants such as Vitamin E and a host of phytonutrients that benefit the immune system. Hazelnuts contain Arginine, an amino acid that relaxes blood vessels, Folate and heart healthy B vitamins. In fact, hazelnuts have the highest concentration of Folate among tree nuts. Folate reduces the risk of neural tube birth defects, and may help to reduce the risk of cardiovascular disease, certain cancers, Alzheimer's disease and depression. Hazelnuts also contain the blood pressure-lowering minerals Calcium, Magnesium and Potassium. Additional research linking nuts to reduced cancer risk has also shown that the amino acid Arginine may inhibit tumor growth and boost immunity.

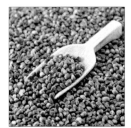

Hemp Seeds: A small complete protein and an excellent source of Omega-3 fatty acids. Contains the following nutrients Vitamins B, C,E, Calcium, Iron, Magnesium, Pantothenic Acid, Phosphorus, Amino Acids, Chlorophyll, Protein: 15%.

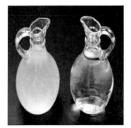

Hydrogenated Oils: Hydrogenated oils are vegetable oils that have been heated to very high temperatures and hardened by injecting hydrogen gas. This process destroys the essential fatty acids (EFA's) and replaces them with unhealthy trans-fatty acids *(cloudy = hydrogenated).*

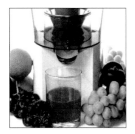

Juicer: A kitchen appliance that extracts juices from vegetables and fruits. A juicer should use a low speed so temperatures will remain low to preserve all the nutrients, enzymes while maximizing yield.

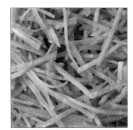

Julienne: A method of cutting vegetables or fruits into matchstick strips.

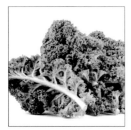

Kale: A cruciferous vegetable with dark green curly leaves. Three varieties are: green kale, red kale, and dinosaur kale (a.k.a. lacinato kale). Great for juicing and green smoothies.

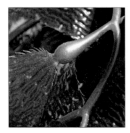

Kelp: a.k.a. "Kombu" Kelp is a very nutrient dense seaweed. Kelp is especially high in Iodine, which must be present for proper glandular function and metabolism. It also contains Iron, Sodium, Phosphorus and Vitamin C, as well as Magnesium and Vitamin P. Kelp is a source of Vitamins A, B1, B2, C, D E, plus Amino Acids. Kelp also makes a popular salt substitute. Because the plant's nutrients come in a natural form, they are easily assimilated by the body.

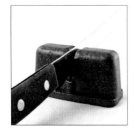

Knife Sharpener: A very essential kitchen appliance. There are 2 types: natural stone and commercial. I highly recommend Chef's Choice for ease of use and price point.

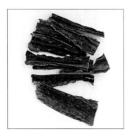

Kombu: Is a Sea Vegetable that is hand harvested wild and sun dried. Eden Kombu is a wide leaf, deep growing sea vegetable that flourishes in the cold Arctic waters of Japan's northernmost island where the best Kombu grows wildly. Only the most tender and central part of the leaf is used because of its mild flavor and pleasing texture. Highly appreciated for it's food value and flavor enhancing characteristics, Kombu has been considered a health food for centuries in Asia. Kombu is an essential ingredient in the delicious Japanese noodle broth, dashi, but can be added to any soup or soup stock to enliven it. Stew it with vegetables. Pickle or deep-fry it. Pan or oven roast and grind into a powder. Kombu makes a tasty and most nourishing table condiment. Sprinkle some on popcorn instead of salt as low-Sodium, delicious variation. A product of Japan.

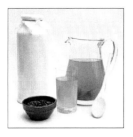

Kombucha: Kombucha Tea (KT) is sugared black tea fermented with a symbiotic culture of acetic acid bacteria and yeasts. It is said to be tea fungus. KT is claimed to have various beneficial health benefits. However, there is very little peer-reviewed scientific evidence available at this time. Some results have shown liver toxicity. I recommend you contact your health care practitioner for guidance.

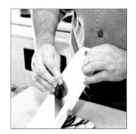

Mandoline: A kitchen utensil with many blades that will slice and julienne fruits and vegetables. Most mandolins of steel will cost you over $100, however the Japanese versions of ceramic are less expensive (under $25) but will only have a single blade for slicing.

Marinate: The act of tenderizing and flavoring by allowing ingredients to soak in oil, dressings, acids (like lemon or lime juice) and salt.

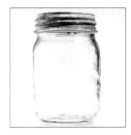

Mason Jars: a.k.a. "canning jars" Glass jars great for storing pantry staples, dressings, sauces, soaking nuts, storing seeds, nuts, and sprouting. I prefer the wide-mouth opening brand with metal screw top lids.

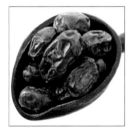

Medjool Dates: Medjool dates are deep amber-brown and have a slightly crinkly skin that shimmers from natural sugar crystals. They taste of rich caramel, hints of wild honey and a touch of cinnamon. Medjools have high carbohydrate and high Potassium levels. Always soak them in purified water and remove the seed before using.

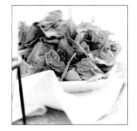

Mesclun Green: Usually mixed and young salad greens consisting of red leaf, baby romaine, oak leaf lettuces arugula, frisée, mâche and radicchio. Always spin greens before using.

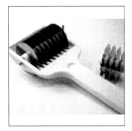

Mincer: A gadget that chops very fine. Onions, garlic, celery, ginger and herbs are generally minced.

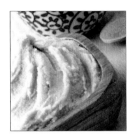

Miso: A paste made with fermented soybean and salt. Miso contains many healthy bacteria and enzymes. Look for organic and unpasteurized located in the refrigeration section. White miso is mild and sweet.

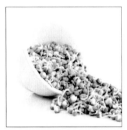

Mung Beans: A medium sized legume used for sprouting. Vitamins A, B, C, E, Calcium, Iron, Magnesium, Potassium, Amino Acids, Protein 20%.

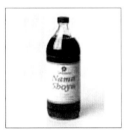

Nama Shoyu: Unpasteurized traditional Japanese soy sauce. Be careful when using in recipes because it *contains wheat.* When using don't use wheat unless it's in the sprouted form. Try using non-wheat versions of Organic Tamari or Bragg's Liquid Aminos. Nama Shoyu can be pricey too!

Nori Sheets: a.k.a. "Nori Seaweed" Green seaweed that comes in very thin sheets and used to make nori rolls for sushi. Be sure to buy the un-toasted kind (brown color).

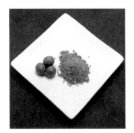

Nutmeg: Nutmeg is the actual seed of the tree. Used in small dosages nutmeg can reduce flatulence, aid digestion, improve the appetite and treat diarrhea, vomiting and nausea. Nutmeg's flavor and fragrance come from oil of myristica, containing myristicin, a poisonous narcotic. Myristicin can cause hallucinations, vomiting, epileptic symptoms and large dosages can cause death. These effects will not be induced, however, even with generous culinary usage.

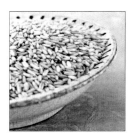

Oat Grouts: Hulled oats, are called oat grouts. They look very much like rye. With a relatively high soluble and insoluble fiber content of 10%, oats are an excellent food in lowering cholesterol and reducing the risk of heart disease. Containing over 4 times the fatty acids of wheat, oats can be considered a high calorie food containing 19% more calories than wheat. One third of those fats are the polyunsaturated type which are required for good health. Oats are also rich in the B vitamins, contain the anti-oxidant vitamin E and oats are mineral rich as well.

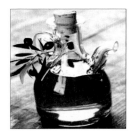

Oils: Flaxseed, Grapeseed, Pistachio, Extra-Virgin Olive Oil, Walnut, Pumpkin, Hazelnut, Almond and Hemp. All of these oils are used in preparing Raw and Living Food. Always store in dark containers and out of the sun or ambient light. This will prevent them from going rancid or being damaged from the sun.

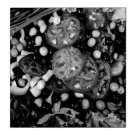

Olives, Greek: a.k.a. "Kalamata Olives" are salt-cured and sun-dried are the best.

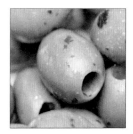

Olives, Green: Raw olives must be cured before they can be eaten, and the curing medium is usually lye, brine, or salt. All of these affect their flavor and texture. So too does the olive's degree of ripeness when it's picked. Green olives are picked while unripe, which makes them denser and bitterer than brown or black olives, which stay on the tree until fully ripened. Opened cans or jars of olives should be refrigerated, but some olives can be stored at room temperature if they're submerged in brine or olive oil.

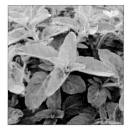

Oregano: Oregano has demonstrated antimicrobial activity against food-borne pathogens such as Listeria monocytogenes. The leaves and flowering stems are strongly antiseptic, antispasmodic, stimulant, and mildly tonic. Oregano is taken by mouth for the treatment of colds, influenza, mild fevers, indigestion, stomach upsets and painful menstruation. It is strongly a sedative and should not be taken in large doses, though mild teas have a soothing effect and aid restful sleep. Used topically, oregano is one of the best herbal antiseptics because of its high thymol content. Hippocrates, the father of medicine, used oregano as an antiseptic as well as a cure for stomach and respiratory ailments.

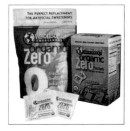

Organic Z® Sweetener: Organic all-natural Zsweet is a blend of erythritol (pronounced ee-rith-ri-tol) and natural fruit extracts as flavor enhancers. Erythritol occurs naturally at low levels in many fruits and such fermented foods as soy sauce, cheese, wine and beer. This proprietary blend is what makes organic all-natural Zsweet taste like sugar—without the sugar worries. Zsweet measures like sugar, and unlike other products, it can be used in baking and cooking, as well as flavoring hot and cold drinks. Allergic side effects can be itching with hives, constipation or diarrhea.

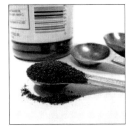

Paprika: Paprika is a spice made from the grinding of dried sweet red or green bell peppers *Capsicum annuum* is mildly flavored and prized for its brilliant red color.

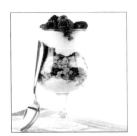

Parfait: A parfait is a dessert normally made by layering cream or ice cream or flavored gelatin dessert with other ingredients such as granola, nuts, sauces or various toppings. In Raw and Living Food nut creams are substituted for ice cream or yogurt. Both are made in a tall, clear glass making all layers visible. The term refers to an ice cream treat similar to a sundae.

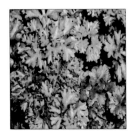

Parsley: The delicious and vibrant taste and wonderful healing properties of parsley are often ignored in its popular role as a table garnish. Highly nutritious, parsley can be found year round in your local supermarket. Parsley is the world's most popular herb. It derives its name from the Greek word meaning "rock celery" (parsley is a relative to celery). It is a biennial plant that will return to the garden year after year once it is established.

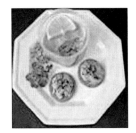

Pâté: A fine or coarsely chopped or ground filling, seasoned with herbs, onions, garlic and salt. Raw and Living Food pâtés are made from nuts, seeds and vegetables.

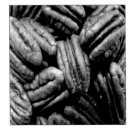

Pecans: Pecans are a good source of protein and unsaturated fats. A diet rich in nuts can lower the risk of gallstones in women. The antioxidants and plant sterols found in pecans reduce high cholesterol by reducing the "bad" LDL cholesterol levels. Pecans are be used for crusts and pâtés in making Raw and Living Food recipes.

Phytonutrients: Natural compounds found in plants that improve the immune system, slow the aging process, and can help prevent heart disease and cancer. (i.e. chlorophyll, lycopene, carotenoids, and bioflavinoids).

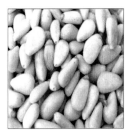

Pine Nuts: a.k.a. "Pignolas or pinons" Pine nuts contain (depending on species) between 10–34% protein. The Stone Pine having the highest content. They are also a source of dietary fiber. When first extracted from the pine cone, they are covered with a hard shell (seed coat), thin in some species, thick in others. The nutrition is stored in the large female tissue that supports the developing embryo in the center. Although a nut in the culinary sense, in the botanical sense pine nuts are seeds.

The shell must be removed before the pine nut can be eaten. Unshelled pine nuts have a long shelf life if kept dry and refrigerated (at –5 to +2 °C); shelled nuts (and unshelled nuts in warm conditions) deteriorate rapidly, becoming rancid within a few weeks or even days in warm humid conditions. They may be lightly toasted by heating in a skillet without any added oil.

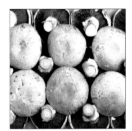

Portabello Mushrooms: These mushrooms are an excellent source of Niacin and a good source of Potassium and Selenium.

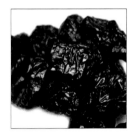

Prunes, Dried: Prune juice contains a natural laxative. Prunes also contain dietary fiber (about 7%, or 0.7 grams per prune). Prunes and prune juice are thus common home remedies for constipation. Prunes have a thick skin covering a juicy pulp—the plum's skin is a source of insoluble fiber, whereas the pulp is a source of soluble fiber. Prunes have a high antioxidant content.

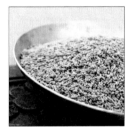

Psyllium: The husks are finely ground into a powder and used in Raw and Living Food as a thickener. You can purchase the coarse ground and finely grind it yourself at home.

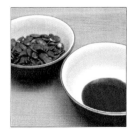

Pumpkin Seed Oil: The seeds are dried and then pressed to release a rich, nutty flavor. The oil is rich in essential fatty acids and is thought to balance hormones.

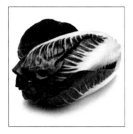

Radicchio is a leaf chicory a.k.a. "Italian chicory". It is grown as a leaf vegetable which usually has white-veined red leaves. It has a bitter and spicy taste, which mellows when it is grilled or roasted. It can also be used to add color and zest to salads.

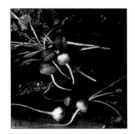

Radish Seeds: A sprouted seed which will add a special "bite" to your recipes. Vitamins A, B, C, E, K, Calcium, Iron, Magnesium, Phosphorus, Potassium, Zinc, Carotene, Amino Acids, Chlorophyll, Trace Elements, Antioxidants, and Protein: 35%.

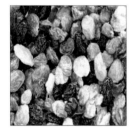

Raisins: Raisins are dried grapes and about 60% sugar by weight, most of which is fructose. They are also high in antioxidants, and are comparable to prunes and apricots in this regard.

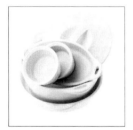

Ramekin: A small ceramic dish approximately 3" in diameter and may hold 6 oz of volume. Ideal for mousses and puddings.

Raw Food: Any unprocessed, unrefined or untreated food group.

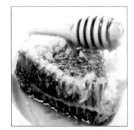

Raw Honey: Honey that has not been processed by heating. Aids stomach and digestion. In digestive disturbances honey is of great value. Honey does not ferment in the stomach because, being an inverted sugar, it is easily absorbed and there is no danger of a bacterial invasion. The flavor of honey excites the appetite and helps digestion. For anemics, dyspeptics, convalescents and the aged, honey is an excellent reconstructive and tonic. In malnutrition, no food or drug can equal it. The laxative value of honey, on account of its lubricating effect, is well known. Its fatty acid content stimulates peristalsis. In gastric catarrh, hyperacidity, gastric and duodenal ulcers and gall bladder diseases, honey is recommended by several eminent gastroenterologists.

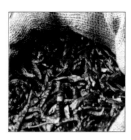

Red Chili Pepper, Dried: The chili pepper, chilli pepper, or chili is the fruit of the plants from the genus Capsicum, which are members of the nightshade family Solanaceae. Even though chilis may be thought of as a vegetable, their culinary usage is, generally, a spice, the part of the plant that is usually harvested is the fruit.The name, which is spelled differently in many regions (chili, chile, or chilli), comes from the Spanish word *chile*. The term chili in most of the world refers exclusively to the smaller, hot types of capsicum. The mild larger types are called bell peppers in the U.S. and Canada.

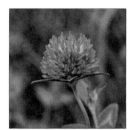

Red Clover Seeds/Sprouts: A small legume usually used for sprouting. Loaded with Vitamins A, B, C, E, K, Calcium, Iron, Magnesium, Phosphorus, Potassium, Zinc, Carotene, Chlorophyll, Amino Acids, Excellent for Women, Trace Elements, and Protein: 35%.

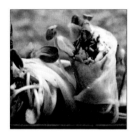

Rice Paper: Rice paper usually refers to paper made from parts of the rice pant, like rice straw or rice flour. However, the term is also loosely used for paper made from or containing other plants like hemp, bamboo, or mulberry. Edible rice paper is used for making fresh summer rolls (also called spring rolls - shown here) or fried spring rolls in Vietnamese cuisine. Ingredients of the food rice paper include white rice flour, tapioca flour, salt and water. The tapioca powder makes the rice paper glutinous and smooth. Kozo is a stiff rice paper is made up to 21.8% cellulose.

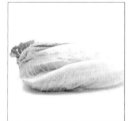

Romaine Hearts: The thick ribs, especially on the older outer leaves, should have a milky fluid which gives the romaine the typically fine-bitter herb taste. Romaine is the standard lettuce used in Caesar salad. Romaine lettuce is often used in the Passover Seder as a type of bitter herb, to symbolize the bitterness inflicted by the Egyptians while the Israelites were slaves in Egypt.

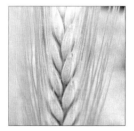

Rye: A grain usually sprouted. Mainly used in salads and dough. Vitamins B, C, E Calcium, Iron, Magnesium, Pantothenic Acid, Phosphorus, Amino Acids, and 15% Protein.

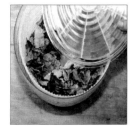

Salad Spinner: A salad spinner is a kitchen tool that washes and spin dries salad greens. It is best to serve salad greens as dry as possible. Spinning also increases the shelf life of your greens.

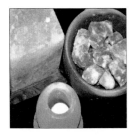

Salt, Unrefined: Himalayan Pink salt, a sun-dried pink salt with a high mineral content. Sea salts come in different textures fine, coarse, light gray, Flower of the Ocean grind (see Celtic Sea Salt® Brand). *CAUTION: Himalayan salt may contain high levels of Fluoride. Check with your healthcare practitioner before using.*

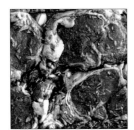

Saturated Fats: Fats that turn solid at room temperature and are usually found in dairy products, red meat, palm oil, coconut oil, cocoa butter, and palm kennel oil. Saturated fats are linked to heart disease.

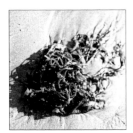

Sea Weed: Seaweed draws an extraordinary wealth of mineral elements from the sea that can account for up to 36% of its dry mass. The mineral macronutrients include Sodium, Calcium, Magnesium, Potassium, Chlorine, Sulfur and Phosphorus; the micronutrients include Iodine, Iron, Zinc, Copper, Selenium, Molybdenum, Fluoride, Manganese, Boron, Nickel and Cobalt.

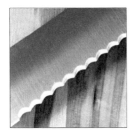

Serrated Knife: A serrated knife is ideal for slicing into foods with thick or tough textures. These knives are also great for cutting tomatoes, peaches, plums, kiwi and the like.

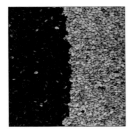

Sesame Seeds, Hulled: Usually sprouted or sprinkled on salads or ground up to make sesame seed flour. Seeds are available in Golden, Beige and Brown. All contain the same nutritional value, however the Brown sesame seed is usually less expensive.

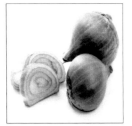

Shallots: Shallots are often thought to be another variety of onion, but they are actually a species of their own. They grow in clusters, where separate bulbs are attached at the base and by loose skins. The shallot has a tapered shape and a fine-textured, coppery skin, which differentiates it from onions. Shallots were first introduced to Europeans during the 12th Century. Crusaders brought them home as "valuable treasure" from the ancient Palestinian city of Ascalon.

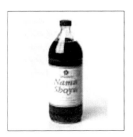

Shoyu: Shoyu is a soy sauce, which is a dark brown liquid made from soya beans that have undergone a fermentation process. Natural shoyu uses a centuries-old method of fermentation which converts hard-to-digest soy proteins, starches and fats into easily absorbed amino acids, simple sugars and fatty acids. Most commercial shoyu is made by a chemical process in which cereals and soybeans are mixed with acids. No other soy sauce in America comes close to this 100% organic, non-GMO Nama Shoyu in flavor or quality. It's the only soy sauce that's aged for four years in cedar kegs by a unique double-brew process, so it can be made with less salt naturally, while still retaining its full-bodied flavor and delicate bouquet. Nama Shoyu is also un-pasteurized. It's full of health-giving live enzymes and beneficial organisms like lactobacillus. **Ingredients**: Organic whole soybeans, mountain spring water, organic whole wheat, sea salt. *Nama Shoyu contains wheat* unlike Tamari or Bragg Liquid Aminos.

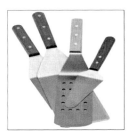

Spatulas: An essential utensil available in many different sizes, shapes, materials and colors. The skinner head is great for removing mixtures from a food processor. The wide metal spatulas and off-set heads are good for removing slices of cake or pies from a pan. Square ones are designed to remove lasagna or some cookies. A triangular one is designed to remove pies and tarts from their pans.

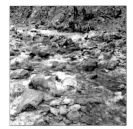

Spring Water: A spring is a point where groundwater flows out of the ground, and is thus where the aquifer surface meets the ground surface. Water issuing from an artesian spring rises to a higher elevation than the top of the confined aquifer from which it issues. When water issues from the ground it may form into a pool or flow downhill, in surface streams. Minerals become dissolved in the water as it moves through the underground rocks. This may give the water flavor and even carbon dioxide bubbles, depending upon the nature of the geology through which it passes. This is why spring water is often bottled and sold as mineral water, although the term is often the subject of deceptive advertising. Springs that contain significant amounts of minerals are sometimes called 'mineral springs'. Springs that contain large amounts of dissolved Sodium salts, mostly Sodium Carbonate are called 'soda springs'.

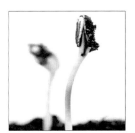

Sprouts: Any nut, seed, grain, legume, or grain that has been soaked in purified water and left to germinate. All sprouts are loaded with vitamins, minerals, amino acids, phytonutrients, protein and amino acids and easily digested.

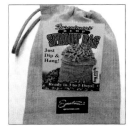

Sprout Bag: A mesh bag in a variety of sizes used to grow sprouts, to strain nuts or to make nut or seed milks.

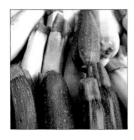

Squash: Summer squash are a subset of squashes that are harvested when immature (while the rind is still tender and edible). All summer squashes are fruits. The name "summer squash" refers to the inability to store these squashes for long periods of time (until winter), unlike winter squashes (Cousa squash, pattypan squash a.k.a. "Scallop squash", yellow crookneck, yellow summer squash and zucchini squash a.k.a. Courgette).

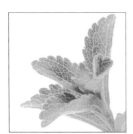

Stevia: a.k.a. "Sweetleaf, Sweet leaf, Sugarleaf or Stevia" *Stevia* has about 150 species and is a member of the sunflower family. It is commonly known as sweetleaf, sweet leaf, sugarleaf, or simply stevia, is widely grown for its sweet leaves. As a sugar substitute, stevia's taste has a slower onset and longer duration than that of sugar, although some of its extracts may have a bitter or licorice-like aftertaste at high concentrations.

With its extracts having up to 300 times the sweetness of sugar, stevia has garnered attention with the rise in demand for low carbohydrate, low-sugar food alternatives. Stevia also has shown promise in medical research for treating such conditions as obesity and high blood pressure. Stevia has a negligible effect on blood glucose, even enhancing glucose tolerance; therefore, it is attractive as a natural sweetener for diabetics and others on carbohydrate-controlled diets.

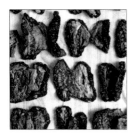

Sun-dried Tomatoes: These are plum tomatoes that have been sun-dried at low temperature. They are a bit chewy in nature and a little tart. Sun-dried tomatoes may be packed in olive oil or dry. Dry ones need to be soaked in purified water at least 30 minutes or longer.

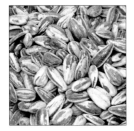

Sunflower Seeds, Raw and/or Hulled: The **sunflower seed** is the fruit of the sunflower. The term "sunflower seed" is actually a misnomer when applied to the seed in its hull. When dehulled, the edible remaining part is called the sunflower kernel.

Commercially, sunflower seeds are usually classified by the pattern on their husks. If the husk is solid black, the seeds are called black oil sunflower seeds. The crops may be referred to as oilseed sunflower crops. These seeds are usually pressed into sunflower oil.

If the husks are striped, the seeds are called striped sunflower seeds or "stripers." Due to their lower oil content, the crops are called non-oilseed sunflower crops. Striped sunflower seeds are primarily used for food.

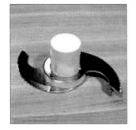

S-Blade: a.k.a. "Spherical Blade" has been designed as a blade for a food processor that can chop, grind, or purée food groups.

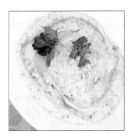

Tahini, Raw: Tahini is sesame paste — meaning it's a paste of ground sesame seeds — used in many Raw and Living Food recipes. Tahini is a major component of hummus and can be fresh or dehydrated. The paste made from black sesame seeds is said to have higher nutritional value than the brown variety.

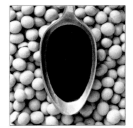

Tamari, Raw: A Japanese soy sauce made without wheat. It has a very rich salty flavor.

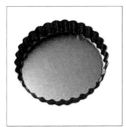

Tart Pan: A pan with fluted edges used in making pastries. They should be Teflon coated for easy removal of the bottom. This feature allows for the easy removal while leaving the crust intact.

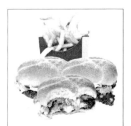

Trans-Fats: These fats are created when vegetable oils are hydrogenated, refined or heated to high temperatures. Most processed foods contain trans-fats which includes snacks, crackers, breads, cookies. Trans-fats create metabolic problems that deposit themselves in the arteries of the body.

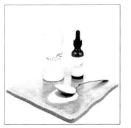

Truvia™: Rebiana comes from the sweet leaf of the stevia plant, native to South America. Dried stevia leaves are steeped in water, similar to making tea. This unlocks the best tasting part of the leaf which is then purified to provide a calorie-free sweet taste. Combined with erythritol, a natural sweetener. Erythritol is a natural sweetener produced by a natual process and is also found in fruits like grapes and pears. It has no after taste like regular stevia. Allergic side effects can be itching with hives or constipation. The author has reason to believe the Rebiana family gene may be a GMO due to reported allergic responses. Use sparingly and with caution. Pure Stevia has been on the market for years with few side effects.

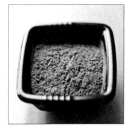 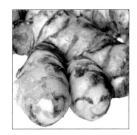

Turmeric: Turmeric is a member of the ginger family. Widely used as an alternative to the more expensive saffron spice.

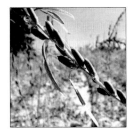

Unhulled Sesame Seeds: Unhulled sesame seeds contain more Calcium than hulled. Brown sesame seeds have the hull intact.

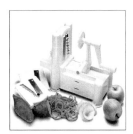 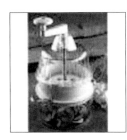 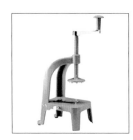

Vegetable Spiral Slicer: a.k.a. "garnishing machine" This gadget makes vegetables like zucchini into a vegetable pasta noodle. Some come with multiple blades. ChefSharynne.com is an affiliate provider.

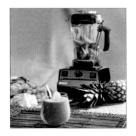

Vita-Mix: Vita-Mix 5200 the newest series of this high-speed, high performance professional-looking blender that makes soups, smoothies, ice cream, sauces and much more in seconds. I personally recommend Vita-Mix. It's my favorite appliance. Eventually this is a must have for raw food preparation. ChefSharynne.com is an affiliate provider.

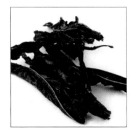

Wakame: a.ka. "alaria" A nutritious seaweed. Wakame is a kelp and looks and tastes like spinach lasagna. Wakame is similar to Kombu and it can be used in many of the same ways, particularly in soup.

Wakame is probably best used in salads, added to soup or broth or used as a topping for other dishes. Soak dried wakame in purified water and it will expand to about ten times in size. Wakame should have the central vein cut out after soaking. It can be ground up in a coffee grinder to turn into a powder. This is an easier way to use when measuring.

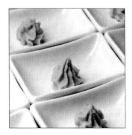 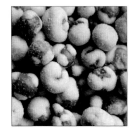

Wasabi: Wasabi is Japanese horseradish. It is most famous in form of a green paste used as condiment for sashimi (raw seafood) and sushi. However, wasabi is also used for many other Japanese dishes. Wasabi is a root vegetable that is grated into a green paste. Wasabi has a strong, hot flavor that dissipates within a few seconds and leaves no burning aftertaste in your mouth.

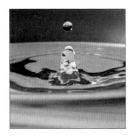

Water: Purified water is critically essential to any Raw and Living Food recipe. It is used in sprouting and washing produce. Any type of water except tap water or softened water is considered "purified". That includes water processing using a Brita or PUR water filter.

My personal choice is alkaline anti-oxidant from Silver Springs Home Delivery service featuring the Real Water E2 Technology. ChefSharynne.com is an affiliate provider.

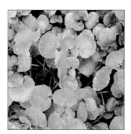

Watercress: *Eating watercress daily can significantly reduce DNA damage to blood cells, which is considered to be an important trigger in the development of cancer,* University of Ulster scientists have revealed. A crispy, salad green with a slightly peppery and bitter flavor.

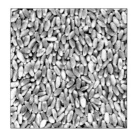

Wheat berries, Hard Winter: a.k.a. "The Nectar of the Gods!" sprouted to make **"wheatgrass".** The ultimate blood purifier, *Wheat Grass Juice is the closest thing there is to blood itself!* Vitamins A, B, C, E, K, Calcium, Chlorophyll, Iron, Lecithin, Magnesium, Pantothenic Acid, Phosphorus, Potassium, Amino Acids, Trace Elements, Protein: up to 30% and much more.

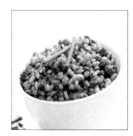

Wheat berries, Spring: Great for sprouting and has Vitamins A, B, C, E, Calcium, Iron, Magnesium, Niacin, Phosphorus, Potassium, All Essential Amino Acids and Protein: 20-25%.

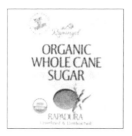 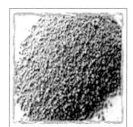

Whole Cane Sugar: USDA Certified Organic Whole Cane Sugar:
'Hand in Hand'-Ecology and Fair-Trade product.
Dried, unrefined, naturally evaporated sugar cane juice.
Processing method retains the original natural vitamins and minerals in the sugar. The harvest is done without the usual "burning-the-dry-leaves-first" technique, but is done all by hand. That means preserving compostable material and no increase of the greenhouse effect. A natural energy source and sweetener. 100% Vegan Sugar.

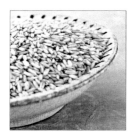

Whole Oat Groats: Unpolished whole kernels; sweet, nutlike flavor; chewy texture. Whole groats are oats before they have been flattened out into the familiar "rolled oats". Make sure they are untreated, as some manufacturers steam them to increase their shelf life.

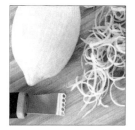

Zest: The outer skin of citrus fruits that is removed using a zester (as shown), peeler or file grater. Be careful not to zest the white pith (meat) as it is very bitter.

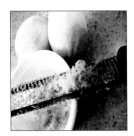

Zester or Microplane: Citrus zester or lemon zester is a kitchen utensil for obtaining zest from lemons and other citrus fruit. A zester is approximately four inches long, with a handle and a curved metal end, the top of which is perforated with a row of round holes with sharpened rims. To operate, the zester is pressed with moderate force against the fruit and drawn across its peel. The rims cut the zest from the pith underneath. The zest is cut into ribbons, one drawn through each hole. Do not go too deep into the rind (pith) as it is bitter in taste. Microplane is great for fine grating of garlic, nutmeg and more.

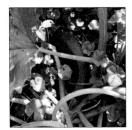

Zucchini: A small summer squash. In the culinary world, zucchini is treated as a vegetable, which means it is usually cooked and presented as a savory dish or accompaniment. Botanically, however, the zucchini is an immature fruit, being the swollen ovary of the female zucchini flower. The male flower grows directly on the stem of the zucchini plant in the leaf axils (where leaf meets stem), on a long stalk, and is slightly smaller than the female. Both flowers are edible, and are often used to dress a meal or garnish. The zucchini vegetable is low in calories and contains good amounts of Folate, Potassium, Vitamin A and 19% of the recommended amounts of Manganese.

LETTUCE LINGO 101

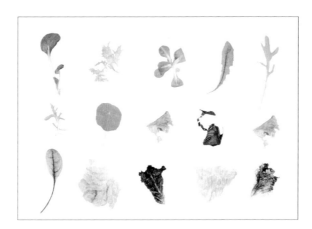

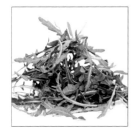

Arugula: Its leaves have a unique, peppery sweet tang, adding pizzazz even to the blandest lettuce varieties. Arugula provides the same flavor impact as onions, but without the aftertaste.

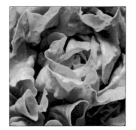

Butterhead: Refers to a family of greens characterized by loosely packed, ruffled leaves and sweetish flavor. Bibb and Boston are two common varieties.

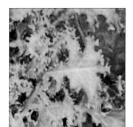

Curly endive: Also known as chicory, it adds a distinctive flair with its loose frilly leaves and bitter taste.

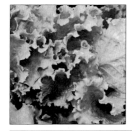

Frisée: Narrow, pale-green leaves with jagged curly edges. Also bitter in taste.

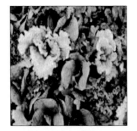

Mesclun: A blend of gourmet greens that refers to the French word for "mixed field greens".

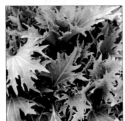

Mizuna: A popular Japanese green with feathery, narrow leaves and a mild mustard flavor.

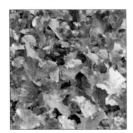

Oak Leaf: Adds a touch of panache, but has limited availability.

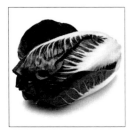

Radicchio: This is more of a cabbage type lettuce with an intense red color and a slightly bitter flavor. Radicchio is generally mixed with other lettuces to enhance the appearance, flavor, and nutritional value of salad.

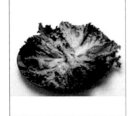

Red or Green Leaf Lettuce: Loose, ruffled leaves that make an excellent salad on their own or a good foundation for a larger creation.

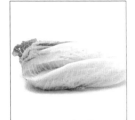

Romaine: A leafy green used most often in the classic Caesar salad.

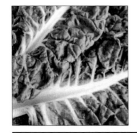 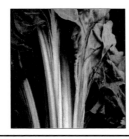

Swiss or Young Chard: Narrow fan-shaped leaves, but usually only the young leaves are used in tossed salads.

COMMON SPICES & THEIR HEALTH BENEFITS

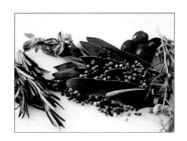

Basil

Good source of beta-carotene
Anti-inflammatory properties
Anti-bacterial properties
Rich in anti-oxidants

Black Pepper

Aids in digestion
Rich in anti-oxidants
Anti-bacterial properties

Cayenne Pepper

Anti-inflammatory
Pain relief
May help prevent ulcers
May assist with weight loss efforts by increasing metabolism
Improves circulation
Decreases mucous production

Cilantro (coriander seeds)

May help control blood sugar
May help cleanse heavy metals from the body
Anti-microbial properties
Rich in phyto-nutrients
May help decrease cholesterol
Aids in digestion

Cinnamon

Boosts brain function
Assists with blood sugar control
Anti-microbial properties
Anti-fungal properties
Anti-clotting properties
Contains Calcium, vitamins and fiber
Aids in digestion

Cumin

Good source of Iron
Anti-carcinogenic properties
Aids in digestion
Believed to be a blood purifier

Curry

Anti-inflammatory
May decrease arthritis pain
May decrease risk of certain types of cancers
May protect against Alzheimer's disease
May decrease cholesterol
May boost brain function

Dill

Good source of Calcium
Anti-bacterial properties
May have anti-carcinogenic properties

Garlic

Anti-bacterial properties
Anti-viral properties
Rich in anti-oxidants
May help decrease cholesterol

Ginger

Aids in digestion
Anti-inflammatory properties
Boosts immune system
May protect against colon cancer

Lemon

Rich source of Vitamin C
Boosts the immune system
Anti-bacterial properties
May be helpful for detoxifying the liver

Mustard

Rich in phyto-nutrients
Anti-inflammatory properties
May improve cardiovascular health
Aids in digestion

Onions

Anti-bacterial properties
May improve respiratory health
May help decrease cholesterol
May improve cardiovascular health

Oregano

Anti-bacterial properties
Rich in anti-oxidants
May assist with respiratory problems
Aids in digestion

Parsley

Improves circulation
Prevents bad breath
Rich in vitamins and minerals
Rich in anti-oxidants
Mild diuretic
May improve kidney function

Peppermint

Aids in digestion
Useful in aromatherapy
Makes a wonderful tea
Rich in phyto-nutrients

Rosemary

Anti-inflammatory properties
Rich in anti-oxidants
Anti-carcinogenic properties
Rich in Vitamin E and minerals
A mild diuretic

May help to detoxify the liver
May improve brain function and memory

Saffron

Aids in digestion
May help with depression
May have anti-carcinogenic properties
Rich in anti-oxidants

Sage

Anti-inflammatory
Anti-microbial properties
Rich in anti-oxidants
May improve brain function and memory

Tarragon

Aids in digestion
May help with insomnia
Anti-inflammatory

Thyme

Anti-bacterial properties
Rich in anti-oxidants
May benefit respiratory health
Improves circulation
Strengthens the immune system

Tumeric

Anti-inflammatory
May decrease arthritis pain
May decrease risk of certain types of cancers
May protect against Alzheimer's disease
May decrease cholesterol
May boost brain function

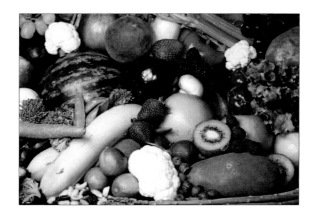

(* An iTunes APP is now available at <u>www.itunes.com</u>.)

JAN: Avocados, bananas, cabbage, cauliflower, mushrooms, pears, potatoes, turnips, winter squash

FEB: Avocados, bananas, broccoli, cabbage, cauliflower, kumquats, mangos, mushrooms, pears, tangerines, winter squash

MAR: Artichokes, asparagus, avocados, bananas, broccoli, grapefruit, kumquats, lettuce, mushrooms, radishes, spinach

APR: Asparagus, bananas, cabbage, chicory escarole, onions, pineapples, radishes, rhubarb, spinach, strawberries

MAY: Asparagus, bananas, celery, papaya, peas, pineapples, potatoes, strawberries, tomatoes, watercress

JUN: Avocados, apricots, bananas, cantaloupe, cherries, corn, cucumbers, figs, green beans, limes, mangos, nectarines, onions, peaches, peas, peppers, pineapples, plums, summer squash

JUL: Apricots, bananas, blueberries, cabbage, cantaloupe, cherries, corn, cucumbers, dill, eggplant, figs, Gravenstein apples, green beans, nectarines, okra, peaches, peppers, prunes, watermelon

AUG: Apples, bananas, beets, berries, cabbage, carrots, corn, cucumbers, dill, eggplant, figs, melons, nectarines, peaches, pears, peppers, plums, potatoes, summer squash, tomatoes

SEP: Apples, bananas, broccoli, carrots, cauliflower, corn, cucumbers, dill, figs, grapes, greens, melons, okra, onions, pears, peppers, potatoes, summer squash

OCT: Apples, bananas, broccoli, grapes, peppers, persimmons, pumpkins, yams

NOV: Apples, bananas, broccoli, cabbage, cauliflower, cranberries, dates, eggplant, mushrooms, pumpkins, sweet potatoes

DEC: Apples, avocados, bananas, grapefruit, lemons, limes, mushrooms, oranges, pears, pineapples, tangerines

COOKING STANDARD MEASUREMENTS

dash   = 1/8 tsp or 8 drops

1 teaspoon   = tsp or "t"
                    = 60 drops

1 tablespoon   = tbs or "T"
                    = 3 tsp

1 ounce   = oz
                    = 2 tbs

1/4 cup   = 2 oz
                    = 4 tbs
                    = 12 tsp
                    = 59 ml

3/4 c   = 6 oz
                    = 12 tbs
                    = 36 tsp

1/3 c   = 2 2/3 oz
                    = 5.3 tbs
                    = 16 tsp
                    = 79 ml
                    = 5 tbs

2/3 c   = 5 1/3 oz
                    = 10.6 tbs
                    = 32 tsp
                    = 158 ml

1/2 c   = 4 oz
                    = 8 tbs
                    = 24 tsp
                    = 118 ml
                    = 8 tbs

1 c   = 8 oz
                    = 16 tbs
                    = 48 tsp
                    = 237 milliliters or ml
                    = 1/2 p (pint)

1/8 c	= 1 oz
	= 2 tbs
	= 6 tsp
	= 30 ml
1/16 c	= 1/2 oz
	= 1 tbs
	= 3 tsp
	= 15 ml
1/2 quart (qt)	= 1 p
	= 2 c
1 qt	= 2 p
	= 4 c
	= 32 oz
1 gallon (gal)	= 4 qt
	= 8 p
	= 16 c
	= 128 oz
1 pound (lb)	= 16 oz
1 gram (gr)	= 1/30 oz
1 ounce	= 30 grams (g or gr)
1 kilo (k)	= 2.2 lbs
1 liter (l)	= 1 q (quart) (approximately) or "qt"
1 tad	= 1/4 tsp
1 pinch	= 1/16 tsp
1 smidgen	= 1/32 tsp

MEDICAL DISCLAIMER

I am not a doctor or a nutritionist, however, I am a certified raw food chef and nutritional educator. The information contained within this book is not intended to diagnose, treat, cure or prevent any disease. Taking natural products should be a decision based on your own personal research and on the understanding of the role that food and food-derived supplements play in health and well being. Natural products should only be used with the advice and support of a qualified natural health care professional. The author is not responsible for the misuse and/or abuse of any products sold or referred to. Website users, previous and future customers who fail to consult their natural health care professional prior to beginning any health and/or fitness regime, assume the risk of any adverse effects.

Thank You

A very special thank you to the authors listed below for their inspiration of this book. These cookbooks are also part of my recommended media in addition to those listed on page 126.

Alt, Carol. *The Raw 50.*
Amsden, Matt. *Rawvolution.*
Boutenko, Sergei and Valya Boutenko. *Fresh—The Ultimate Live Food.*
Boutenko, Victoria. *12 Steps to Raw Foods.*
Boutenko, Victoria. *Green for Life.*
Bragg, Patricia. *Vegetarian Health Recipes.*
Cobb, Brenda. *The Living Food Lifestyle.*
Cohen, Alissa. *Living on Live Food.*
Cornbleet, Jennifer. *Raw Food Made Easy.*
Elliott, Angela. *Alive in 5.*
Hamlyn, *Juices & Smoothies.*
Juliano, *RAW—The Uncook Book.*
Kenney, Matthew and Sarma Melngalis. *Raw Food—Real World.*
Olivier, Suzannah. *Fresh & Raw.*
Patenaude, Frederic. *Instant Raw Sensations.*
Phyo, Ani. *Ani's Raw Food Kitchen.*
Reinfeld, Mark and Bo Rinaldi. *Idiots' Guide to Eating Raw.*
Rhio, *Hooked on Raw.*
Rufell, Wendy. *The Raw Transformation.*
Schneider, Joyce and Robert Schneider, MD. *Chocolate Too! Diet.*
Shannon, Nomi. *The Raw Gourmet.*
Soria, Cherie. *Angel Foods, The Raw Revolution.*
The Boutenko Family. *Raw Family.*
Trotter, Charlie and Roxanne Klein. *Raw.*

RECOMMENDED MEDIA

Books

Living on Live Food—Alissa Cohen
Living Foods for Optimal Health—Brian Clement
Diet for a New America—John Robbins
God's Way To Ultimate Health—Rev. George Malkmus
Raw Secrets—Frederic Patenaude
Eat to Live—Dr. Joel Fuhrman
The China Project—T. Colin Campbell, PhD.
Your Right to Know—Andrew Kimbrell

Videos

"Living On Live Food"—Alissa Cohen
"Eating - Plus" (This is awesome!)—Rave Diet/Michael Anderson
Any of Dr. Day's videos (www.drday.com)
"Miraculous Self-Healing Body"—Hallelujah Acres

Web Sites

www.shazzie.com — Some spectacular raw transformation stories
www.rawfoodchef.com — When you're ready to learn more about Raw and Living Food
www.rawfoodinfo.com — Rhio's site: recipes, resources, and directories

Networking

— Find a raw buddy: Someone that you can share resources and recipes with, provide support, encouragement and account-ability.

—Raw Food Meet-up or Potluck Groups: If you don't have one in your area, START ONE!

ABOUT THE AUTHOR

Sharynne Gambrell-Frazer is the Owner and Founder of www.ChefSharynne.com and www.SharynneFrazer.com.

She is a Barnes & Noble best-selling author, caterer, educator, and public speaker on Healthy Lifestyles, located in Las Vegas, Nevada.

Her client list is impressive:

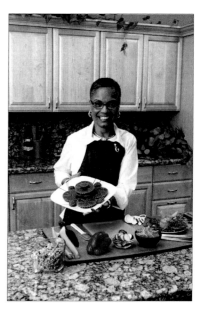

- Whole Foods Market
- Trader Joe
- Internal Health Wellness
- Breast Center at Sunrise Hospital
- St. Rose Hospital
- Barbara Greenspun-Womens Center
- Tupperware
- Anthem-Sun City
- Tropical Smoothie Café-Hawaii
- Hawaii Wellness Retreats-Hawaii
- Olelo Community Television-Hawaii
- Bullivant Houser Bailey, PC
- Zippy's Restaurant-Hawaii
- Unity Church of Hawaii

- Wine the Experience-Hawaii
- Senator Mike Gabbard-Hawaii
- Arbonne International-Hawaii
- Powerhouse Gym-Hawaii
- The Amie Jo Radio Show
- College Park Rehab Center
- Global Health Chiropractic-Hawaii
- Back 2 Health Chiropractic-Hawaii
- Vim N Vigor Organics-Hawaii
- Henderson OB-GYN
- Curves
- Siena Homeowners Association
- Bosch Kitchen Store
- Miss Kapialani 2009-Hawaii

Ms. Frazer is a Certified Living Food Chef and Teacher—honors she obtained from studying with Alissa Cohen and her "Living on Live Food" program in Kittery, Maine. Alissa Cohen is one of the five top Living Food gurus and teachers in the world.

A passion for advising and helping people to practice a healthy lifestyle has developed into a thriving business for Ms. Frazer, whose high-spirited, outgoing personality and knowledge of the importance of eating well continues to enhance and advance her career.

Ms. Frazer graduated from the School of Certified Laboratory Technologists and was one of seven students selected statewide, in Ohio, by the American Society of Clinical Pathology. Her education led to the position of Head Laboratory Technician for Marvin A. Levy, M.D. and Allan S. Silverman, M.D.—private practice "physicians to the stars" in Beverly Hills, California. She continued her studies and graduated salutatorian as a Certified Surgical Technologist through the Association Surgical Technologist.

Ms. Frazer has an extensive thirty-year medical background with studies in Anatomy, Physiology, Hematology, Blood Banking, Urinalysis, Chemistry, Bacteriology, Clinical Pathology, Robotic and Automated Blood Chemistry, X-ray Technology and Histology.

She started BIO-P.M. Services, Inc., a Bio-medical company serving the Greater Los Angeles area that performed routine bio-medical laboratory tests using medical robotics. Clients included Kaiser Permanente, Genetech, Smith-Kline Beecham, San Diego U.S. Naval Hospital, National Institute of Health, Nicholls Institute and Genetics Institute. Ms. Frazer opened a similar company, Sharell Corporation, located in Las Vegas. Clients included American Pathology Laboratories plus the clients mentioned above. American Pathology Laboratories is now Quest Diagnostics—the largest privately-owned blood chemistry facility in the State of Nevada.

Ms. Frazer is a graduate of the Living Light Culinary Arts Institute in Ft. Bragg, California, where she studied under the institute's Director, Cherie Soria. Cherie is an internationally-known, thirty-year raw food pioneer, author and speaker. Ms. Frazer is an Associate Instructor with the Living Light Culinary Arts Institute.

THANK YOU FOR PURCHASING MY BOOK!

With your purchase you are entitled to a complimentary ten-minute telephone coaching call. Please email me so we can set up your appointment: info@ChefSharynne.com.

I hope I have inspired you to arm yourself with information and become an informed consumer and natural health advocate. Write down your experiences and share them with others. Who knows—it may end up being YOUR first book!

Thank you for allowing me to share my Passion with YOU!

Enjoy Your JOURNEY!

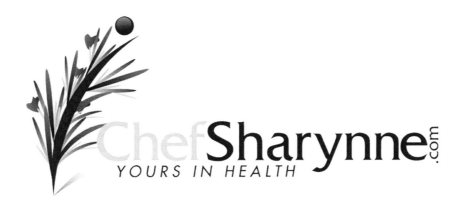